Inhibitory Control Training - A Multidisciplinary Approach

Edited by Sara Palermo and Massimo Bartoli

Published in London, United Kingdom

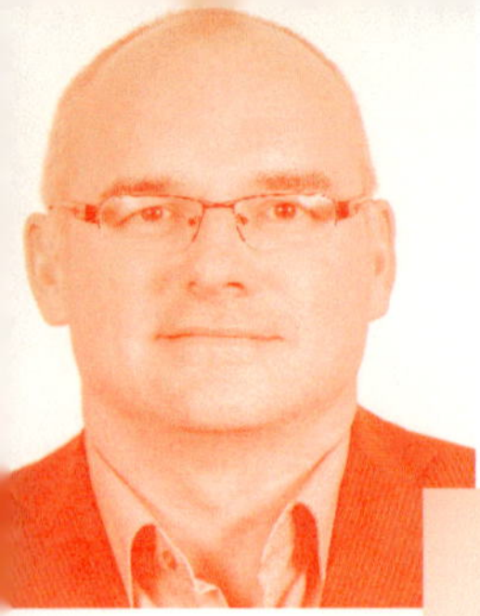
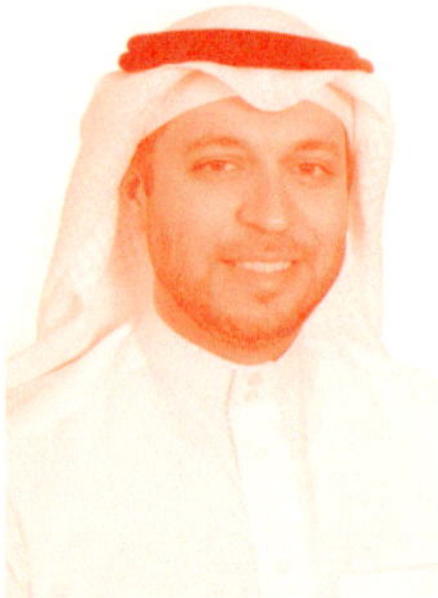
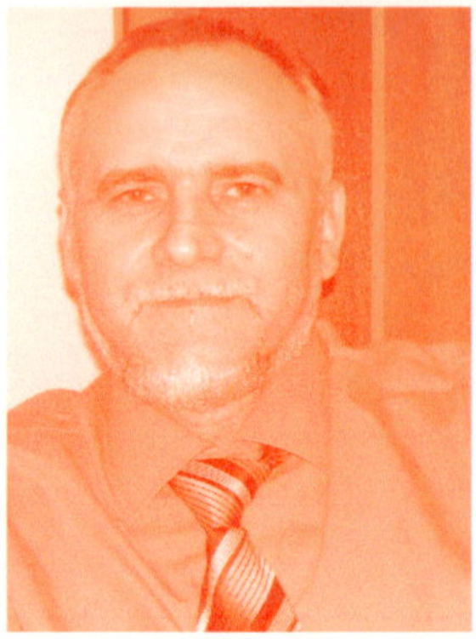
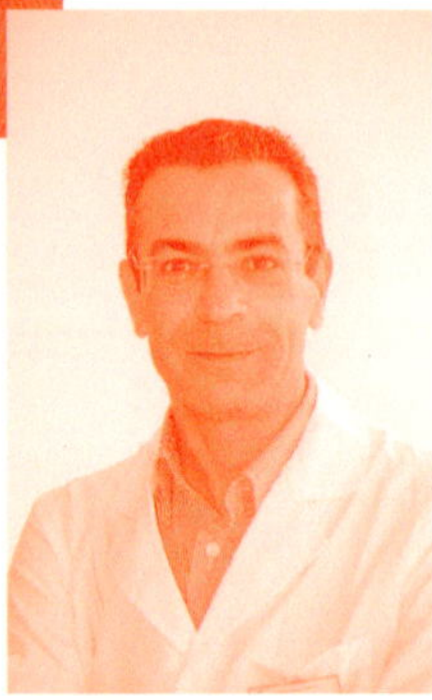
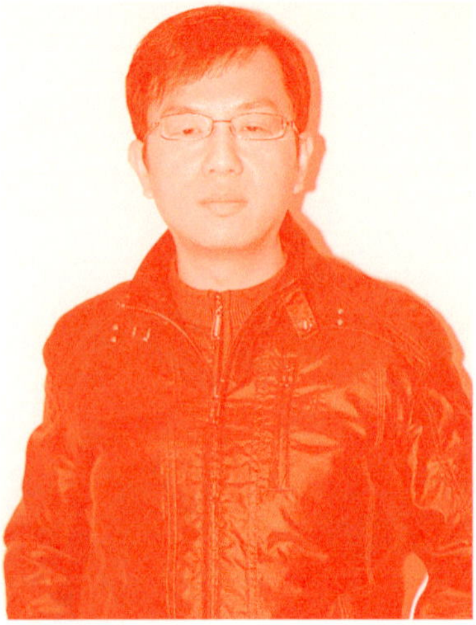
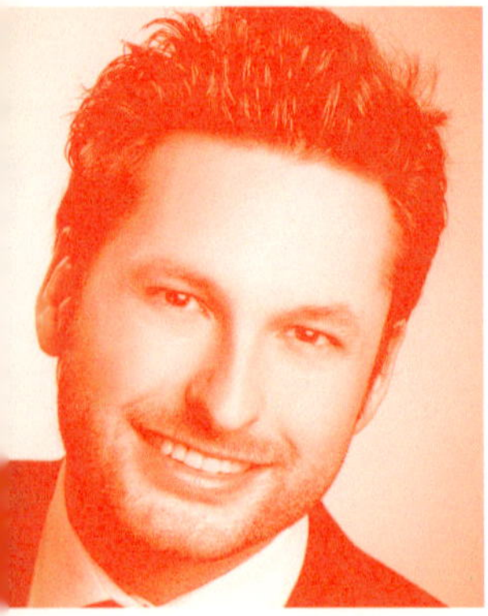
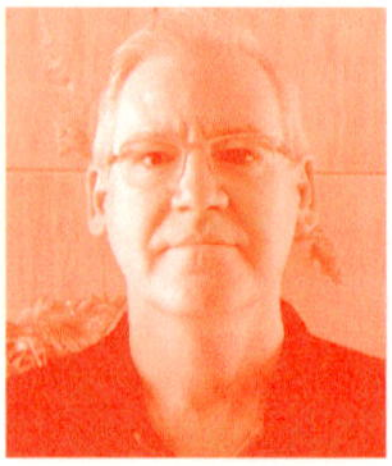

IntechOpen

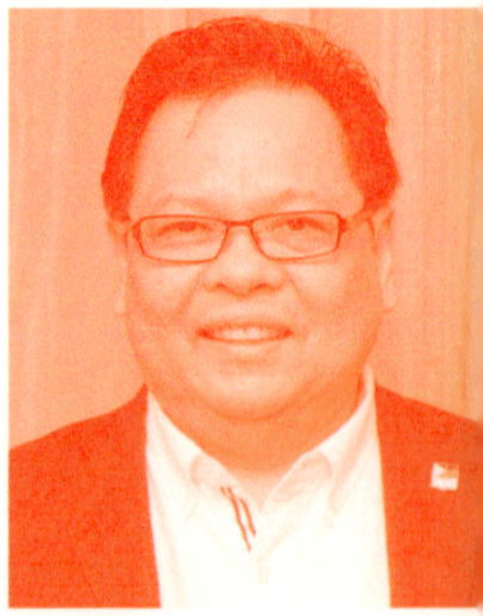
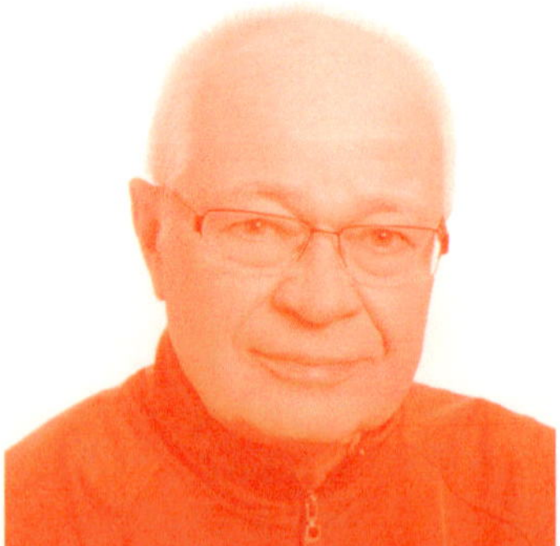
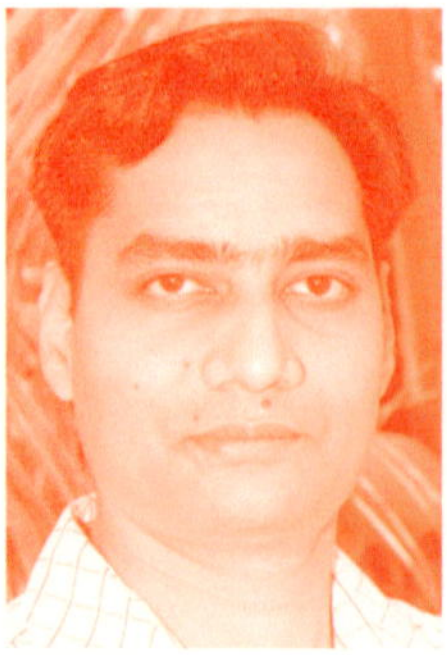
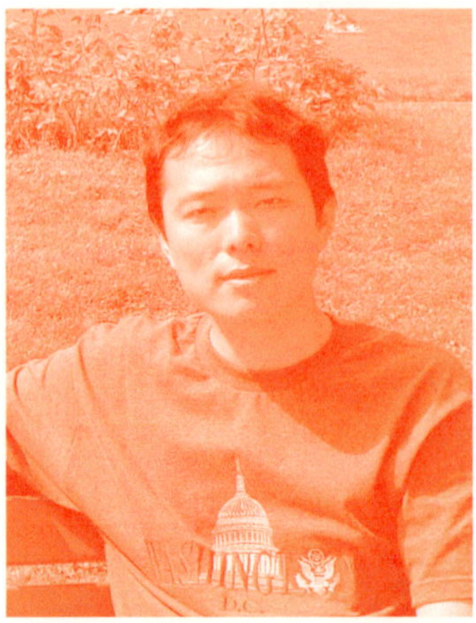
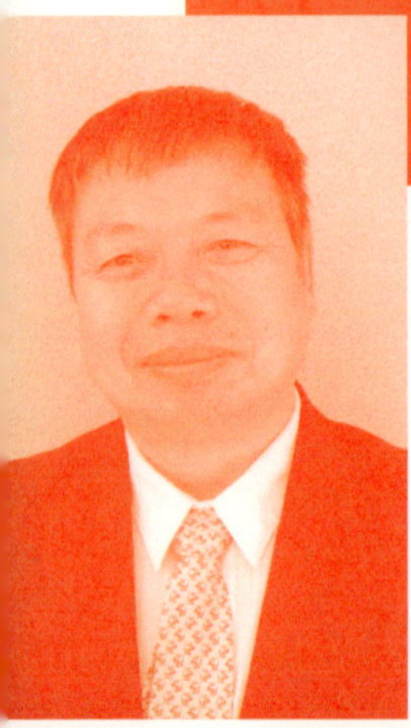
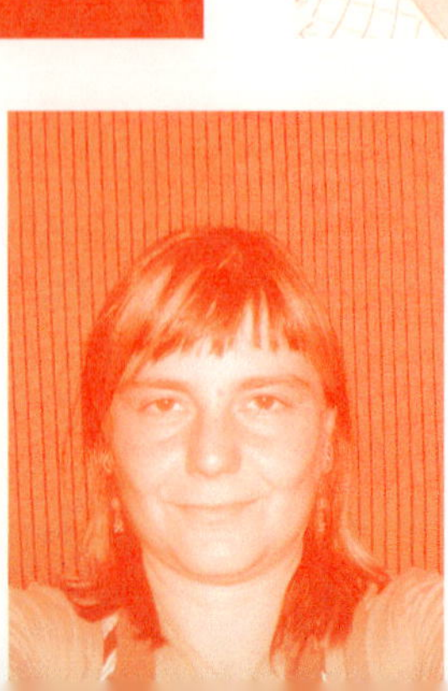

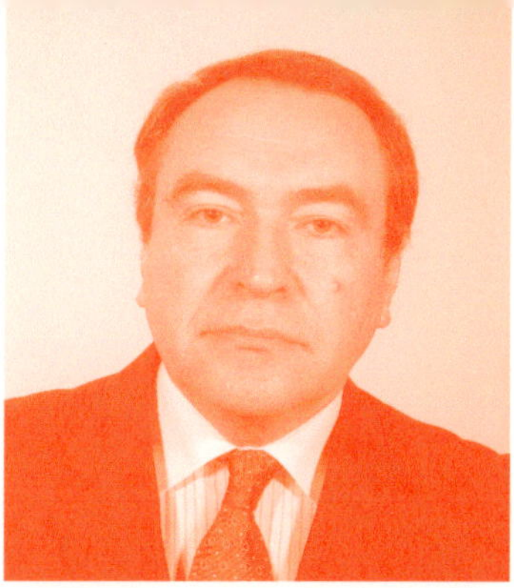
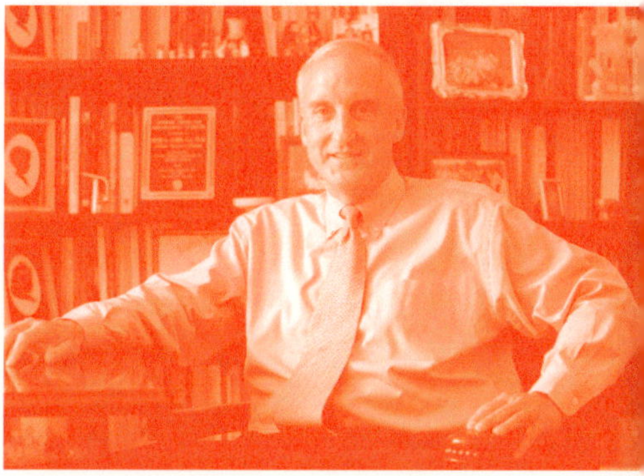
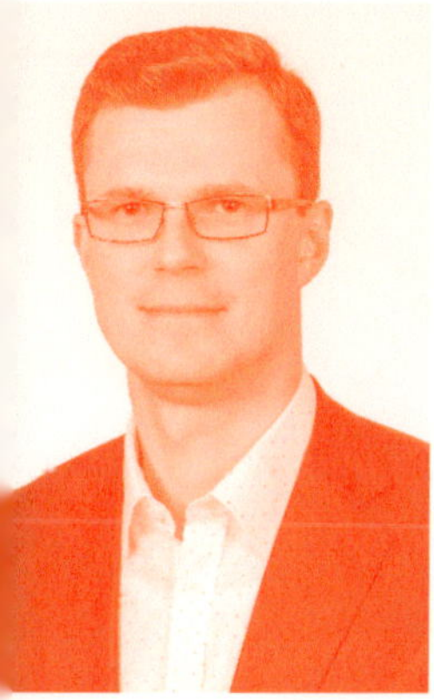
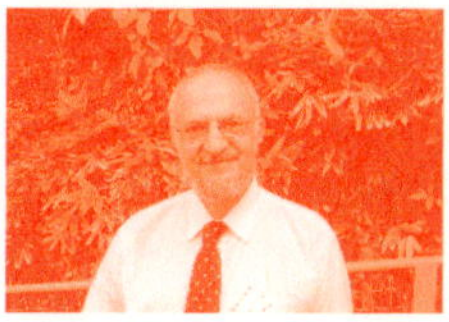
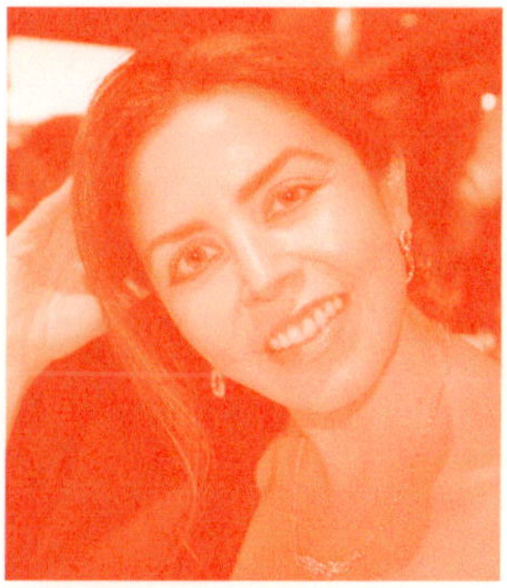

Supporting open minds since 2005

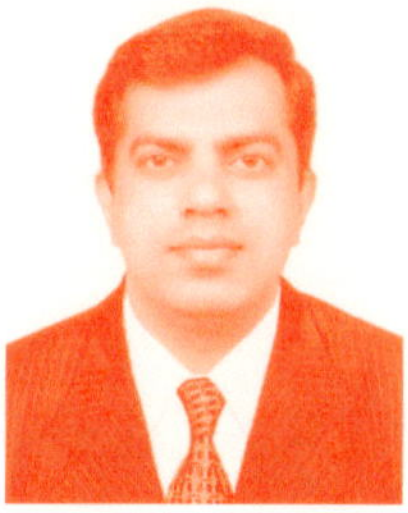
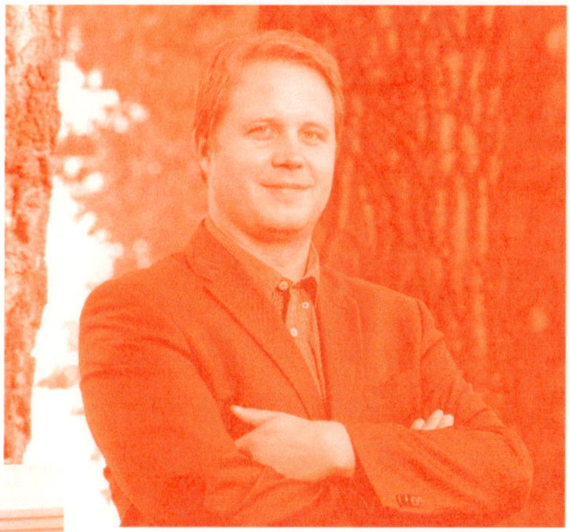
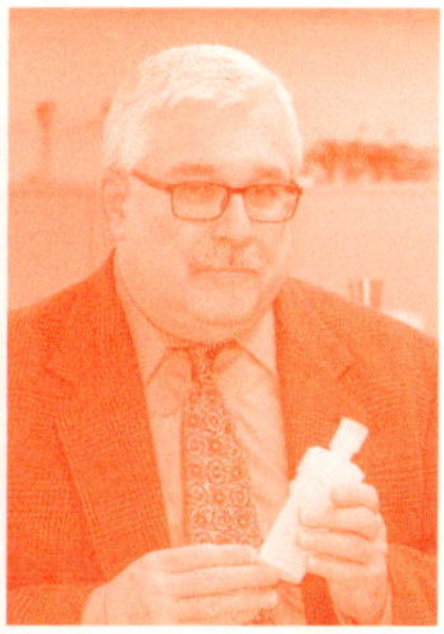
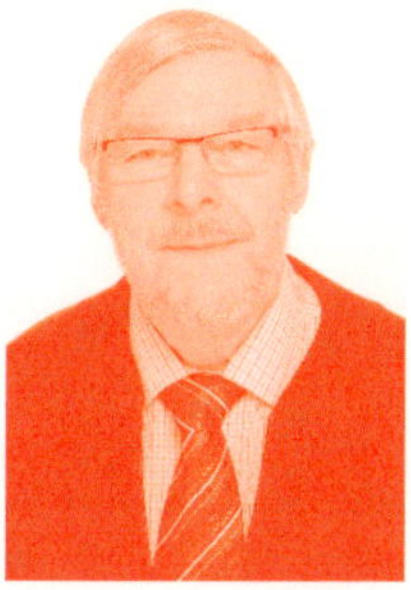
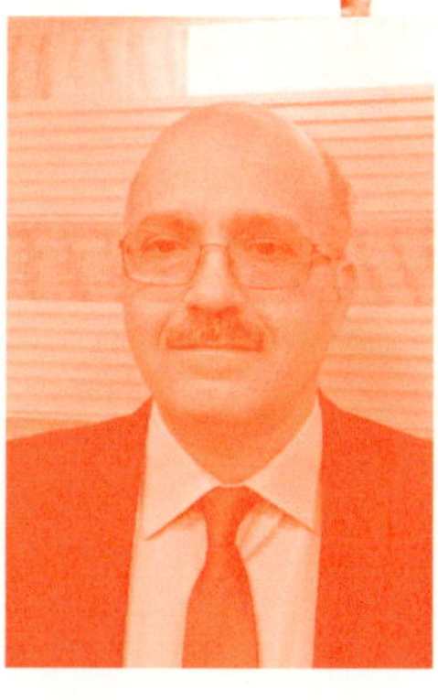
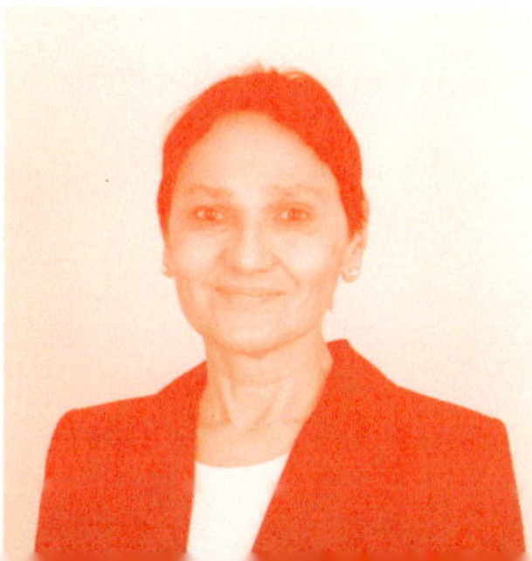
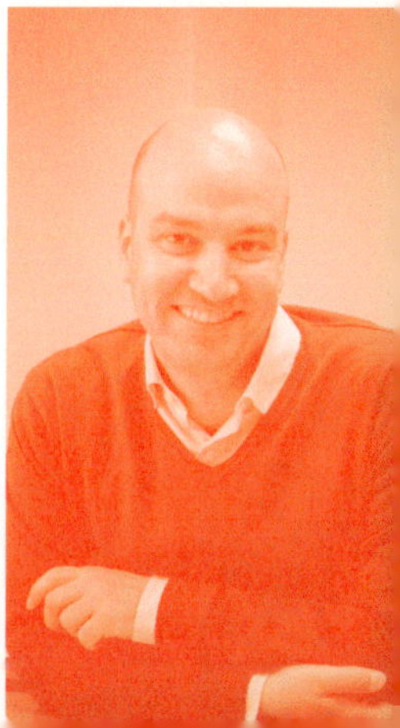

Inhibitory Control Training - A Multidisciplinary Approach
http://dx.doi.org/10.5772/intechopen.82899
Edited by Sara Palermo and Massimo Bartoli

Contributors
Concepción Vinader-Caerols, Santiago Monleon, Xavier Noel, Patricia Gorman Barry, Marilyn Welsh, Jared M. Greenberg, Erin Baker, Qingyang Liu, Rong Huang, Jean Gagnon, Wan Seo Kim, Joyce Quansah, Claudia Gonzalez, Robbin Gibb, Frank Robertson

First published in London, United Kingdom, 2020 by IntechOpen
IntechOpen is the global imprint of INTECHOPEN LIMITED, registered in England and Wales, registration number: 11086078, 7th floor, 10 Lower Thames Street, London, EC3R 6AF, United Kingdom
Printed in Croatia

British Library Cataloguing-in-Publication Data
A catalogue record for this book is available from the British Library

Additional hard and PDF copies can be obtained from orders@intechopen.com

Inhibitory Control Training - A Multidisciplinary Approach
Edited by Sara Palermo and Massimo Bartoli
p. cm.
Print ISBN 978-1-78985-981-2
Online ISBN 978-1-78985-982-9
eBook (PDF) ISBN 978-1-83880-527-2

Meet the editors

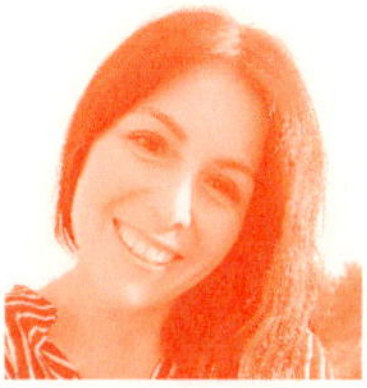

Sara Palermo has her MSc in Clinical and Community Psychology and her PhD in Experimental Neuroscience. She is a research member of the "Center for the Study of Movement Disorders" and the "Placebo Responses Mapping Group" at the Department of Neuroscience (UNITO), and a research member of the "Neuropsychology of cognitive impairment and CNS degenerative diseases group" at the Department of Psychology (UNITO). She is member of the Italian Society of Neuropsychology, the Italian Association of Psychogeriatrics, the Italian Autonomous Association adhering to SIN for dementias, and the International Society for Interdisciplinary Placebo Studies. She is a member of the European Innovation Partnership on Active and Healthy Aging, for which she is involved in the Action Group "Functional decline and frailty".

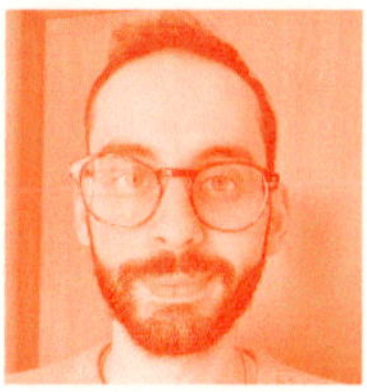

Massimo Bartoli has his MSc in Criminal and Forensic Psychology with a postgraduate specialization in Psychopathology and Forensic Neuropsychology at the University of Padua (Italy). He has worked with the Italian Society of Sexual Psychopathology on several research projects concerning the psychopathological and neuropsychological characteristics of sexual offenders and the assessment of static and dynamic risk factors of sex-crime recidivism. Currently, he is a PhD student in Cognitive Neuroscience at the University of Turin. One of the aims of his PhD project is to investigate the possible association between executive dysfunctions and behavioral and functional aspects, including the legal capacity in subjects with mild and major neurocognitive disorders, and criminal recidivism.

Contents

Preface

Inhibitory control (including response-inhibition and interference-control) is a critical neurocognitive skill for navigating cognitive, social, and emotional challenges. It rapidly increases during the preschool period and is important for early cognitive development, as it is a crucial component of executive functioning, self-regulation, and impulsivity. Inhibitory control (IC) involves the ability to suppress automatic but incorrect responses or to resist interference from distracting stimuli, to reduce a non-target's impact on ongoing information processing. Deficits in IC are a hallmark of psychopathology. Reduced inhibitory control may manifest itself at a *motor level* (e.g. hyperactivity); an *attentional level* (distractibility and difficulty paying attention); and at a *behavioral level* (e.g. impulsive conducts).

Inhibitory control training (ICT) is a novel intervention in which participants learn to associate appetitive cues with inhibition of behavior. Indeed, it can be conceptualized as the ability to stop, change, or delay a behavioral response.

It is a promising approach in the treatment of appetitive behavior, considered as the active, goal-seeking, and exploratory phase of behavior that precedes the more stereotyped consummatory act. Upon reaching the goal, appetitive behavior normally ceases. In some cases, this does not happen.

This book aims to bring together knowledge on the topic, considering research, clinical trials, and the forensic field of intervention. Authors offer original contributions to develop new perspectives in the field of inhibitory control training research thanks to the originality of their ideas, theories, research, scientific results, and discussions.

The first chapter is on the fundamental question of the nature of inhibitory control during the early childhood years, considering the impact of culture and environment on its development. Authors investigate a relevant issue that is the improvement of the capacity to monitor and control thoughts and behaviors by means of ICT. Research on the effects of musical education on executive functions development has generated increasing interest across the scientific community. The second chapter deals with the effects of musical training on inhibitory control in adolescence. The scientific community pays attention also to the link between addiction, developmental deficit, and the appearance of neurocognitive-behavioral dysfunctions. The third chapter investigates inter-individual variations within the addiction group in respect to neurobiological mechanisms of addiction and the risk associated with a limited response inhibition. Authors detail response inhibition theories and methods, summarizing cognitive training intervention in the context of addictive behaviors as well as brain stimulation and neurofeedback techniques. The fourth chapter investigates a relevant issue that is how to improve deductive reasoning abilities thanks to a metacognitive training procedure on executive functions in secondary school students suffering from binge drinking. The fifth chapter outlines alterations of executive functions and inhibitory control following (and aggravated) by conditions of individual and social vulnerability. Authors discuss a critical thinking skills intervention, BrainWise, which is designed to teach inhibitory and self-regulation skills to children, youth, and adults. The last chapter focuses on executive determinants of aggressive behavior and its manifestations. Inhibitory control dysfunctions have implications for refining and targeting training and rehabilitation programs aimed at reducing aggressive behavior. Authors propose the possibility of intervening in terms of ICT. The chapter reviews studies that highlight the relevance of initiating a shift of paradigm from a one-person-cerebral functioning model to a social interactive-cerebral functioning model of impulsive aggression.

Considering the above, this book can be considered a fruitful synopsis of perspectives, methods, empirical evidences, and international references. Moreover, it represents an extraordinary opportunity to outline new horizons on ICT clinical applications.

No man is free who is not master of himself.
(Epictetus)

Control is the source of strategic power.
(Noam Chomsky)

Sara Palermo, PhD and Massimo Bartoli, MSc
Department of Psychology,
University of Turin,
Italy

Chapter 1

A View from the Start: A Review of Inhibitory Control Training in Early Childhood

Erin Ruth Baker, Qingyang Liu and Rong Huang

Abstract

Young children's capacity to monitor and control their thoughts and behaviors is influenced largely by inhibitory control, which grows rapidly during this age due to brain maturation. This capacity has important implications for children's development, including academic and social outcomes, and has been shown to be influenced by culture and exposure to adverse life events such as poverty. Research suggests that this capacity, importantly, may be largely trainable, with appropriate training programs.

Keywords: early childhood, executive function, cross-cultural, low-income

1. Introduction

During the childhood years and into adolescence, the brain grows tremendously, causing a significant change in cognitive capacities. In later years of childhood and adolescence, many of the neurological changes correspond with advancements in perspective taking and reasoning; however, evidence from the early childhood years suggests that these changes more closely align with advancements in inhibitory control and executive functions more broadly [1, 2]. However, there are distinct developmental changes which inform our understanding of inhibitory control and which merit further discussion. Regardless, these developmental changes have profound impacts on children's development overall, including academic and social outcomes. It is important to recognize, however, that children's capacities to inhibit a prepotent response have been shown to vary by culture, as well as exposure to early adverse life events, and therefore a consideration of environment should be included when attempting to conduct research in this area or when making important policy or curriculum decisions. Nevertheless, research which utilizes inhibitory control (IC) training specifically within the early childhood ages demonstrates positive results, with more intensive training yielding more promising results.

2. Nature of inhibitory control during the early childhood years

Research has consistently demonstrated that the preschool years are a developmental time during which children experience profound growth in their ability to inhibit an unwanted response [3]. Younger preschool-age children are more likely to perseverate in their errors across multiple trials [4] by repeating a maladaptive behavior—for instance, a child who continues to shout out in class instead of raising their hand—whereas this pattern declines markedly by age 4. Similarly, 3-year-old children demonstrate an ability to inhibit an automatic prepotent response on a Simon Says task (e.g., Go/NoGo task [5]: children are trained to respond to one stimulus and are trained not to respond to a similar stimulus; see **Table 1**) for roughly one in four trials, in comparison to 4-year-old children who were successful on roughly 9 out of 10 trials [6]. Moreover, the impacts of inhibitory control on children's cognitive capacities also seem to change as a function of age. For instance, younger preschool-age children's inhibitory control capacities strongly predict their problem-solving strategy use and performance; however, older preschool-age children's problem solving is better explained by their working memory capacities (see **Table 1**) rather than their inhibitory control abilities [7]. Relatedly, the development patterns of IC growth may not be limited to simply greater accuracy on relatively straightforward tasks. Older preschool-age children perform with greater success on more complicated tasks of IC than their younger peers [1], which may indicate that using multiple, progressive tasks when assessing IC may reveal important developmental patterns not captured by using a single task or by using

Key terms	Definitions
Executive functions (EF)	The constellation of foundation cognitive capacities, such as inhibitory control, working memory, and attention, which allow for later emergence of reasoning and problem solving
Inhibitory control (IC)	The cognitive capacity to inhibit a prepotent, automatic behavioral response
Working memory	A cognitive system for temporarily storing and managing information that is necessary for undertaking complex cognitive tasks
Theory of mind (ToM)	The understanding that others have mental states such as beliefs, desires, etc., which can vary from person to person or within one person over time
Go/NoGo task	Children are trained to respond to one stimulus (e.g., "Go" stimuli) and are trained not to respond to a similar stimulus ("NoGo" stimuli). This task measures behavioral inhibition
Day/Night Stroop task	Children are trained and must complete trials in which they say the word "night" when presented with an image of a sun on a white background and say "day" when presented with an image of a moon on a dark background. This task involves both behavioral inhibition and cognitive interference
Cognitive interference/interference control	It refers to attempts to suppress interference from competing stimuli. The response time of an IC task is usually considered as a measure of cognitive interference
Behavioral inhibition	It requires suppressing a behavioral response for a more optimal response. Cognitive interference and behavioral inhibition are two aspects of IC
Electroencephalogram (EEG)	A neurological testing that allows researchers to precisely measure brain activity during the behavioral tasks, which provides for a more complete examination and consideration of IC as a cognitive capacity
Inhibitory control training	A designed intervention that includes a training process which aimed at improving IC

Table 1.
A summary of definitions of the major concepts and techniques.

multiple similar tasks. Overall, the findings on early childhood IC show robust and dramatic growth, particularly during the childhood years.

Although researchers agree on the tremendous growth of IC during this developmental age, there persists disagreement as to the specific nature of IC, and executive functions, during this time. Executive functions (EF) refer to the constellation of foundational cognitive capacities, such as inhibitory control, working memory, and attention [1], which allow for later emergence of reasoning and problem solving. In middle childhood and beyond, these executive function capacities can be considered as increasingly discrete processing mechanisms; however, during early childhood, these patterns remain more nebulous, and studies using confirmatory factor analysis have shown developmental differences in factor emergence and persistent factor unification into the childhood years. For instance, during the preschool years (broadly, ages 3 years to 6 years), studies using multiple assessments of inhibitory control, attention, and working memory yield a single unitary construct of executive function or inhibition generally [8–12], whereas studies of middle childhood have discerned multiple discrete factors, including working memory and attention shifting [13], and this trend continues and expands into later childhood and adolescence (see [14]).

The prevailing argument is that tasks of IC during the early childhood years necessitate activation of multiple other components of EF. take, for instance, the Day/Night Stroop task (see [15]; **Table 1**) in which a child is trained and must complete trials in which they say the word "night" when presented with an image of a sun on a white background and say "day" when presented with an image of a moon on a dark background. In this task, IC is typically measured by accuracy, with measurements of response time frequently included as well. This task clearly requires the child to inhibit the automatic response of verbalizing the association they have made between the sun and it being daytime, or between the moon being present during nighttime, and thus is inarguably a task of IC. However, some argue that this task measures additional facets of EF simply by the nature of the task. For instance, a child must have sustained attention throughout the assessment, and if the child loses focus for even a moment, the measurement of response time could be conflated, leading some scholars to argue that the attentional component of EF predicts IC [3, 16]. Similarly, the child must work to keep the rules of the moon/day and sun/night matching in the forefront of their mind during the assessment, and if they do not, then the accuracy measure could be conflated with working memory. Many researchers have argued, therefore, that the various EF components are highly integrated during the early childhood years and that these components emerge as more distinct with age and experience [1, 14].

As shown by the previous example, it is difficult for researchers to disentangle the various components of EF, from a measurement perspective, in early childhood. Researchers' understanding and measurement of inhibitory control during the early childhood years should therefore be sensitive to the developmental nature of such phenomena and should perhaps consider using indices of a variety of executive function capacities. However, as described previously [14], a common conceptualization of EF in the early childhood literature seems to imply that EF and IC are analogous at this development time (e.g., [17]) or that IC developmentally precedes other domains of EF (e.g., [16]). Although IC contributes largely to early childhood EF, as demonstrated in the previous example, it may be problematic to consider these as synonymous. One argument in support of this claim is that children's task performance on EF tasks most closely replicates issues of IC—that is, a child will persist in making prepotent errors, a classic demonstration of immature IC, while also activating other areas of EF, such as attention, working memory, etc. Although several arguments have been proposed to counter the position of equivocating EF with IC, most pertinent to the current chapter may be that IC itself may be multidimensional. Referring again to the aforementioned example, many researchers consider response time in the Day-Night Stroop task to be a measure of *cognitive interference* (sometimes referred to as interference control), which refers to attempts to suppress interference from competing stimuli, in contrast to *behavioral inhibition* which requires suppressing a behavioral response for a more optimal response [18, 19]. That is, the construct of inhibitory control as it pertains to developmental changes during the early childhood years requires both the cognitive power to limit attention to distractor stimuli and the behavioral power to engage an appropriate response.

Turning to developing an appreciation for the role of IC for holistic development, the capacity for IC has important implications in terms of development across a number of domains [20]. For instance, although IC has been shown to predict children's academic achievement generally throughout the childhood years [21], strong IC consistently predicts more proficient mathematical knowledge [16, 22–24] and numerical strategy use [25]. Moreover, IC has been implicated in children's emergent literacy proficiency [16, 24] and language development [26]. The development of IC during the early childhood years additionally has profound implications for children's social and emotional development [27], such as the emergence and development of social perspective taking [28], problem solving and emotional control [27], and suppressing disruptive behaviors and aggression [11]. As such, IC should be considered by researchers and practitioners alike for the implications this capacity may hold across areas of maladaptive academic and social development.

Research methodologies employed for assessing IC during the early childhood years can vary considerably, and each assessment offers a wealth of strengths yet, as mentioned previously, may be incomplete on its own. Therefore, much of the research studies in this area use more than one type of assessment or multiple assessments with considerable methodological overlap. An important consideration in measurement of IC, indeed of any cognitive faculty, during the early childhood years is the developmental appropriateness of the task (see [8], for review). For instance, children in this age range are often concurrently experiencing emerging literacy skills and are often not yet proficient readers; therefore, it would be inappropriate to use a task which requires even low reading requirements, as such a task would likely require a cognitive load too great to allow for successful task completion. Moreover, such a task when used with an emerging reader would result in contaminated measurement in that task performance may indicate a lack of understanding the rules of the task, the lack of proficiency in reading, or inhibitory control. Similarly, tasks to be used on a study of early childhood should be rather straightforward, without overly complicated instructions or numerous steps. Therefore, much of the research studies in the area of inhibitory control that focus on early child development utilize tasks or games which require no reading, with simple instructions provided to the child verbally and repeated if necessary, and these tasks typically include a generous training time to ensure that the child understands and can perform the task.

Many of the commonly employed tasks resemble that of the Day/Night Stroop task [15, 29] and the Go/NoGo task [1, 5, 19, 30], both of which were described in the previous paragraphs. Importantly, these two tasks differ in terms of cognitive interference with regard to the expectations for children's behavioral responses. Specifically, the Day/Night Stroop task involves embedded rule use, thus requires children to produce a verbal response to multiple stimuli, and therefore requires that the children process and act on multiple rules (i.e., if moon, then "day," but if sun, then "night"), whereas the Go/NoGo task only requires a behavioral response to a single stimulus (e.g., if "Simon Says," then response; if not, then no response).

This distinction has led some to argue that the Day/Night Stroop task may be more complex particularly for younger children than other tasks, and therefore performance on this and similar tasks may be indicative of greater IC capacities compared with Go/NoGo tasks (see, e.g., [31, 32]).

Consistent with the recommendation noted previously regarding the need to use multiple indices of IC when attempting to correctly assess children's capacities, many researchers employ the use of neurological testing, such as an electroencephalogram (EEG), in concert with a behavioral task, such as the Go/NoGo task (e.g., [30]). Using neurological measurement, such as EEG, allows researchers to precisely measure brain activity during the behavioral tasks, which provides for a more complete examination and consideration of IC as a cognitive capacity particularly from a developmental perspective. That is, as the brain is experiencing tremendous growth during the early childhood years, it is important to capture how such physical growth corresponds with cognitive growth, and this is perhaps best done by measuring neural activity during a cognitive task.

Overall, EF generally, and inhibitory control specifically, undergoes dramatic growth during the preschool years, which has important implications for their development overall [1, 2]. Although EF is discernable as more discrete constructs in later ages of development, this has not been consistently demonstrated during the early childhood years [8–12], and thus researchers should consider possibly utilizing multiple tasks, including neurological assessments if possible [30], to provide a more comprehensive understanding of IC during the early childhood years.

2.1 Impacts of culture and environment on young children's inhibitory control development

Consistent with other cross-cultural research which shows variation in the timing and emergence of children's cognitive capacities (e.g., [33]), evidence of IC development from non-Western societies is not entirely consistent with that of Western societies, suggesting that children's inhibitory control may be impacted by cultural and environmental factors [34]. For instance, a variety of studies comparing Chinese samples to Western samples may suggest that preschool-age children reared in Chinese cultures outperform their US counterparts on tasks of IC [34, 35], which has also been found in other non-Western cultures (e.g., Japan [36]). Importantly, comparing samples of non-Western cultures from African and Latin American communities [37] as well as cultures which share both Western and Eastern ideals (i.e., Turkey [38]) to Western has not yielded differences by culture. Overall, the cross-cultural research on IC development in early childhood may indicate that although there is a large universality in terms of IC development, cultural and societal mores may cause differences in children's IC and development more broadly.

Moreover, in terms of implications of the cross-cultural research for child development more broadly, in Western cultures IC has been consistently shown to predict theory of mind (i.e., the understanding that others have mental states such as beliefs, desires, etc., which can vary from person to person or within one person over time [39]) particularly during the early childhood years [31], which holds implications for children's social competence during early childhood and beyond; however, this predictive relation between IC and theory of mind has not consistently been demonstrated in cross-cultural samples to the same degree as in Western samples [40]. For example, a recent meta-analysis discussed that although IC and EF generally did predict theory of mind and mental state understanding across cultures, the strength of this prediction was weaker among studies assessing East Asian samples than several Western samples, including the USA, Canada, and Europe [31].

Other environmental factors, such as exposure to poverty or low socioeconomic opportunity, have also been shown to impact children's cognitive development, including the development of EF during the early childhood years, with children from low-income families generally underperforming their more affluent peers [41, 42]; however, the recent work has turned to focus on the adaptive strengths of children raised in environments with higher rates of adversity [43]. For example, although children from low-income families have demonstrated less accuracy on a Go/NoGo task, they did not perform more slowly on the task [44]. Moreover, children from low-income families performed less accurately on a simple working memory task than with peers, but these group differences were eliminated when the task was made to be more complex [44]. A similar finding has been shown for children who have experienced familial trauma, and this may be true even when considering the impacts of poverty exposure. Children who have been reported as experiencing family trauma, as assessed by indices of post-traumatic stress disorder (PTSD), showed poorer global EF than non-traumatized children [45]; however, the effect size was weaker for IC task performance than other types of EF, such as working memory and processing speed. This may suggest that children who experience familial trauma may develop adaptive responses to their environments which allow them to inhibit prepotent responses as indicated by the IC task performance.

Similar to the pattern of IC mediating the impact of culture on early childhood competence, it may be that environmental exposure to poverty and adversity may additionally impact other areas of children's development. Academic achievement and behavioral regulatory faculties are more strongly predicted by IC task performance for children from more affluent family backgrounds, for example, than their less affluent peers [46]. Additionally, among children attending a federally funded educational program for low-income families and their children, children with stronger IC performance were rated by their teachers as having better socio-emotional faculties and showed fewer internalizing behaviors (e.g., indications of anxiety and depression) than their low-income peers who performed less well on IC tasks [47, 48]. Children who experience other types of environmental adversity, such as children who experience violence or maltreatment at home, show similar patterns of poorer academic achievement and school adjustment, yet this relation is additionally explained by children's IC [49]. In sum, although children who experience adverse early life events, or are raised in low-income families and neighborhoods, have shown to differ from more traditional samples in terms of academic achievement and socio-emotional competencies, these discrepancies may be explained by young children's emerging IC faculties. Therefore, these children may show marked improvements in EF capacities, as well as other positive outcomes such as improved academic achievement, with IC training.

2.2 Inhibitory control training in early childhood and implications for development

Efforts in establishing inhibitory control as an effective tool for cognitive improvements have proven successful across the life span [50]. Moreover, as the early childhood years are an important time for the development of EF generally, and IC specifically, as previously discussed, this developmental age range is ideal for examining the possible power of IC training. Several studies have examined the impacts of IC training on child outcomes, and these studies consistently yield positive findings [19, 21, 50–56].

Importantly, the outcomes of IC training have been shown to vary considerably based on the types of training. Studies have shown, for example, the training of more global EF capacities rather than IC specifically (e.g., [53, 55]) may be successful in expanding cognitive performance across a wide range of tasks. This aligns with the aforementioned discussion of the entanglement of multiple components of EF during early childhood (i.e., that many factor analytic studies have shown that in the early childhood years the distinct components of EF, such as working memory and IC, may not be as separately discernable as evidenced during the later years of development [8–12]). To test this, some researchers have attempted to gauge the effectiveness of IC training compared with training in other areas of EF, such as working memory; for instance, children who received 5 weeks of computerized IC training, compared with a group who received a parallel program of working memory training, showed improvements in task performance for the task on which they received training; however these improvements did not transfer to other tasks of EF [55]. Limited transfer effects have been reported elsewhere as well, such as children showing increased performance on methodologically and structurally similar tasks as to the training task, but not other tasks [51], although this increase in performance was sustained over many months. However, other research has shown considerable transfer effects, such as children showing enhanced reasoning abilities after training on a Go/NoGo task [19] and children, adolescents, and adults showing enhanced perspective-taking capacities after receiving IC training [50].

Other types of training have also shown to be successful in improving EF performance. Having children engage in reflective metacognition regarding their performance on difficult cognitive tasks, such as their performance in the Day/Night Stroop task, has shown to be effective in enhancing their performance on that task even compared with more traditional training procedures, such as practice and corrective feedback [54]. Additionally, training on language skills can have a positive impact on children's IC, as such trainings require engaging in multiple components of EF (e.g., sustained attention), as well as IC specifically [57] such as by requiring the child to use the correct term for a specific item within a larger category of items. This aligns with the espoused conceptualization of early childhood IC as profoundly entangled within EF and is consistent with other research on EF trainings more broadly. For instance, children who received 12 sessions over 4 weeks of training that included working memory, IC, and cognitive flexibility showed significant improvements across a range of EF capacities, and these effects transferred to other areas of children's cognition as well [58].

Additionally, outcomes of IC training may yield important changes at the level of neuronal and brain activity [54], which may not necessarily correspond with immediate changes in behavior. For instance, studies have shown that children who received an 8-week program of training which targeted children's IC, working memory, and planning ability found that, for children who received the training, neural activity levels changed in the corresponding brain regions as expected; however children's task performance after the training did not differ significantly from their pre-training performance [30]. Other studies have found that a single training session of metacognitive reflection about controlling impulsive behaviors may lead to decreased activation of the brain region responsible for processing conflicting information, which may indicate a lessened likelihood to process the information as conflicting, and therefore possibly indicating better adaptation in integrating new rule schemes [54].

Moreover, the positive impacts of receiving EF training have been found effective for children from low-income families as well. For instance, one study showed that when classrooms serving low-income families implemented a full year of an EF training that included a broad range of EF skills deeply integrated into the classroom curriculum, compared with classrooms that had no such program, children who received the training outperformed children in the control group on both simple and advanced tasks [52]. Indeed, children in the control group showed a decline in task performance for the more advanced tasks, which was not found for children who received the training. What's more, the program was so successful that the control condition was not allowed to repeat, by request of the school, as the teachers and parents noted such profound change in terms of academics and student behavior that the school refused to continue the project without full implementation of the program in all classrooms. In concert with findings from more traditional samples which included less intensive training, these outcomes would indicate that children from low-income families might be an especially important area for future research, given the overwhelming strength of the results.

Although studies using IC training with children of incarcerated parents, or children who have experienced abuse or neglect, were not revealed during the current literature search, the previously discussed research of IC training during early childhood could be extended to these populations [45]. For instance, research on treatment approaches for anxiety and depression (common outcomes of trauma) with adults has shown that training individuals to develop better self-regulatory executive processes, such as attention, have shown promising results (see [45] for discussion). Given that children's EF faculties are more nebulous and entangled than adults, it stands to reason that such approaches would yield additionally promising results during the early childhood years.

Moreover, such intervention approaches might be promising for researchers working in clinical settings. For instance, mindfulness training approaches that capitalize on EF processes, such as attentional focus, for children with anxiety have proven effective in reducing anxiety symptomology [59]. Such training has proven effective for children from low-income families as well [60], with positive effects extending beyond advanced EF development to include positive socio-emotional and behavioral changes as well. However, much of the research in this area has been conducted with older children, and examinations of the promise of mindfulness training during the early childhood years may not yet exist. This may be an important area for future research, as the implications for positive outcomes may be more robust with earlier intervention.

Overall, findings with regard to improving child outcomes during the early childhood years as they relate to IC training suggest that IC training may be effective to varying degrees. Although a few studies showed limited transfer effects, the most promising findings come from studies which implemented a broader EF training program rather than those which utilized specific IC training. Additionally, research studies with longer training programs, such as the 1-year program discussed above, yield stronger effects in terms of global child outcomes than did shorter programs. Studies involving brain imaging have also shown positive outcomes in terms of changes in brain activity, indicating that such training may be important for effecting long-term change.

3. Conclusions

The cognitive capacity to inhibit a prepotent, automatic response grows tremendously during the early childhood years corresponding with and as a function of profound brain development taking place at this time [1, 2]. At later ages, this cognitive ability is rather distinct from other foundational cognitive capacities, such as attention and working memory; however, considerable research suggests that during early childhood these distinctions are less clear, leading many researchers to consider and research EF as a more global function at this age [8–14].

Research which focuses on IC during the early childhood years typically utilizes simple, game-like tasks which require brief or no verbal response, and researchers typically utilize a variety of tasks which may assess various areas of EF, including the Day/Night Stroop task [15, 29] and the Go/NoGo task [1, 5, 19, 30]. Importantly, and with regard for the important growth occurring at this age in specific brain regions, many researchers use these tasks in combination with brain imaging [30], providing important insights into developmental changes taking place in brain and neuronal activity.

Importantly, the current chapter includes much literature on EF broadly rather than focusing specifically on IC and IC training. Although this is consistent with the current conceptualization of IC during this developmental time within the literature, this may have resulted in certain findings and trainings being included in the current discussion with which some researchers may disagree. Additionally, the current chapter focuses narrowly on a specific developmental window and thus is not representative of the research on IC across childhood.

For transparency, the literature review for the current chapter used the following databases: Google Scholar, ScienceDirect, and Web of Science. The keywords were executive function, inhibitory control (training), working memory, sustained attention, cognitive development, self-regulation, preschoolers, early childhood, children, cross-cultural, and risk population. Specifically, inhibitory control is a broad term in the research procedure, which has been expanded and is not limited to the executive function and cognitive development [61]. For ease of understanding, an at-risk population was defined as any potential risk factors (i.e., poverty or low income, neighborhood violence, family violence, family maltreatment, low social status, low education background, rural area). However, and as is the case with many reviews, the current chapter does not include findings from unpublished works, and thus the positive support for IC training as discussed here may be an artifact of publication bias.

Nevertheless, in creating IC training programs, much of the research has shown positive outcomes across a variety of training programs; however, as is to be expected, more promising and profound results accompany programs with more intensive training with longer durations [50–58]. Such training programs have proven effective across cultures and changes in the environment [52], including children from low-income backgrounds and children who have experienced profound early adverse life events. Although little research to date has examined IC training during early childhood in clinical samples, extending from the work discussed in this chapter, it would follow that IC training broadly, and perhaps mindfulness training specifically, may yield positive outcomes across domains.

Conflict of interest

The authors declare there is no conflict of interest.

Author details

Erin Ruth Baker*, Qingyang Liu and Rong Huang
University at Albany, State University of New York, Albany, NY, United States

*Address all correspondence to: erbaker@albany.edu

References

[1] Anderson PJ, Reidy N. Assessing executive function in preschoolers. Neuropsychology Review. 2012;**22**(4): 345-360

[2] Munakata Y, Herd SA, Chatham CH, Depue BE, Banich MT, O'Reilly RC. A unified framework for inhibitory control. Trends in Cognitive Sciences. 2011;**15**(10):453-459

[3] Reck SG, Hund AM. Sustained attention and age predict inhibitory control during early childhood. Journal of Experimental Child Psychology. 2011;**108**(3):504-512

[4] Diamond A, Taylor C. Development of an aspect of executive control: Development of the abilities to remember what I said and to "Do as I say, not as I do". Developmental Psychobiology. 1996;**29**(4):315-334

[5] Luria AR. Higher Cortical Functions in Man. Berlin: Springer Science & Business Media; 2012

[6] Jones LB, Rothbart MK, Posner MI. Development of executive attention in preschool children. Developmental Science. 2003;**6**(5):498-504

[7] Senn TE, Espy KA, Kaufmann PM. Using path analysis to understand executive function organization in preschool children. Developmental Neuropsychology. 2004;**26**(1):445-464

[8] Garon N, Bryson SE, Smith IM. Executive function in preschoolers: a review using an integrative framework. Psychological Bulletin. 2008;**134**(1):31

[9] Hughes C, Ensor R, Wilson A, Graham A. Tracking executive function across the transition to school: A latent variable approach. Developmental Neuropsychology. 2009;**35**(1):20-36

[10] Miyake A, Friedman NP, Emerson MJ, Witzki AH, Howerter A, Wager TD. The unity and diversity of executive functions and their contributions to complex "frontal lobe" tasks: A latent variable analysis. Cognitive Psychology. 2000;**41**(1):49-100

[11] Raaijmakers MA, Smidts DP, Sergeant JA, Maassen GH, Posthumus JA, Van Engeland H, et al. Executive functions in preschool children with aggressive behavior: Impairments in inhibitory control. Journal of Abnormal Child Psychology. 2008;**36**(7):1097

[12] Wiebe SA, Espy KA, Charak D. Using confirmatory factor analysis to understand executive control in preschool children: I. Latent structure. Developmental Psychology. 2008;**44**(2):575

[13] van der Sluis S, de Jong PF, van der Leij A. Executive functioning in children, and its relations with reasoning, reading, and arithmetic. Intelligence. 2007;**35**(5):427-449

[14] Zelazo PD, Müller U. Executive function in typical and atypical development. In: Blackwell Handbook of Childhood Cognitive Development. Oxford, England: Blackwell Publishers; 2008. pp. 445-469

[15] Gerstadt CL, Hong YJ, Diamond A. The relationship between cognition and action: performance of children 312-7 years old on a stroop-like day-night test. Cognition. 1994;**53**(2):129-153

[16] Blair C, Razza RP. Relating effortful control, executive function, and false belief understanding to emerging math and literacy ability in kindergarten. Child Development. 2007;**78**(2):647-663

[17] Kirkham NZ, Cruess L, Diamond A. Helping children apply their knowledge to their behavior on a

dimension-switching task. Developmental Science. 2003;**6**(5):449-467

[18] Friedman NP, Miyake A. The relations among inhibition and interference control functions: a latent-variable analysis. Journal of Experimental Psychology. General. 2004;**133**(1):101

[19] Liu Q, Zhu X, Ziegler A, Shi J. The effects of inhibitory control training for preschoolers on reasoning ability and neural activity. Scientific Reports. 2015;**5**:14200

[20] Carlson SM. Developmentally sensitive measures of executive function in preschool children. Developmental Neuropsychology. 2005;**28**(2):595-616

[21] Allan NP, Hume LE, Allan DM, Farrington AL, Lonigan CJ. Relations between inhibitory control and the development of academic skills in preschool and kindergarten: A meta-analysis. Developmental Psychology. 2014;**50**(10):2368

[22] Bull R, Scerif G. Executive functioning as a predictor of children's mathematics ability: Inhibition, switching, and working memory. Developmental Neuropsychology. 2001;**19**(3):273-293

[23] Espy KA, McDiarmid MM, Cwik MF, Stalets MM, Hamby A, Senn TE. The contribution of executive functions to emergent mathematic skills in preschool children. Developmental Neuropsychology. 2004;**26**(1):465-486

[24] McClelland MM, Cameron CE, Connor CM, Farris CL, Jewkes AM, Morrison FJ. Links between behavioral regulation and preschoolers' literacy, vocabulary, and math skills. Developmental Psychology. 2007;**43**(4):947

[25] Fuhs MW, McNeil NM. ANS acuity and mathematics ability in preschoolers from low-income homes: Contributions of inhibitory control. Developmental Science. 2013;**16**(1):136-148

[26] Barac R, Bialystok E. Bilingual effects on cognitive and linguistic development: Role of language, cultural background, and education. Child Development. 2012;**83**(2):413-422

[27] Fishburn FA, Hlutkowsky CO, Bemis LM, Huppert TJ, Wakschlag LS, Perlman SB. Irritability uniquely predicts prefrontal cortex activation during preschool inhibitory control among all temperament domains: A LASSO approach. NeuroImage. 2019;**184**:68-77

[28] Carlson SM, Moses LJ, Hix HR. The role of inhibitory processes in young children's difficulties with deception and false belief. Child Development. 1998;**69**(3):672-691

[29] Baker ER, Jensen CJ, Tisak MS. A closer examination of aggressive subtypes in early childhood: contributions of executive function and single-parent status. Early Child Development and Care. 2019;**189**(5):733-746

[30] Pietto ML, Giovannetti F, Segretin MS, Belloli LM, Lopez-Rosenfeld M, Goldin AP, et al. Enhancement of inhibitory control in a sample of preschoolers from poor homes after cognitive training in a kindergarten setting: Cognitive and ERP evidence. Trends in Neuroscience and Education. 2018;**13**:34-42

[31] Devine RT, Hughes C. Relations between false belief understanding and executive function in early childhood: A meta-analysis. Child Development. 2014;**85**(5):1777-1794

[32] Zelazo PD, Jacques S. Children's rule use: Representation, reflection, and cognitive control. Annals of Child Development. 1997;**12**:119-176

[33] Shahaeian A. Sibling, family, and social influences on children's theory of mind understanding: New evidence from diverse intracultural samples. Journal of Cross-Cultural Psychology. 2015;**46**(6):805-820

[34] Sabbagh MA, Xu F, Carlson SM, Moses LJ, Lee K. The development of executive functioning and theory of mind: A comparison of Chinese and US preschoolers. Psychological Science. 2006;**17**(1):74-81

[35] Lan X, Legare CH, Ponitz CC, Li S, Morrison FJ. Investigating the links between the subcomponents of executive function and academic achievement: A cross-cultural analysis of Chinese and American preschoolers. Journal of Experimental Child Psychology. 2011;**108**(3):677-692

[36] Kuwabara M, Smith LB. Cross-cultural differences in cognitive development: Attention to relations and objects. Journal of Experimental Child Psychology. 2012;**113**(1):20-35

[37] Chasiotis A, Kiessling F, Hofer J, Campos D. Theory of mind and inhibitory control in three cultures: Conflict inhibition predicts false belief understanding in Germany, Costa Rica and Cameroon. International Journal of Behavioral Development. 2006;**30**(3):249-260

[38] Orta IM, Corapci F, Yagmurlu B, Aksan N. The mediational role of effortful control and emotional dysregulation in the link between maternal responsiveness and Turkish preschoolers' social competency and externalizing symptoms. Infant and Child Development. 2013;**22**(5):459-479

[39] Baker ER, Jensen CJ, Moeyaert M, Bordoff S. Socioeconomic status and early childhood aggression: moderation by theory of mind for relational, but not physical, aggression. Early Child Development and Care. 2018:1-5

[40] Duh S, Paik JH, Miller PH, Gluck SC, Li H, Himelfarb I. Theory of mind and executive function in Chinese preschool children. Developmental Psychology. 2016;**52**(4):582

[41] Farah MJ, Shera DM, Savage JH, Betancourt L, Giannetta JM, Brodsky NL, et al. Childhood poverty: Specific associations with neuro-cognitive development. Brain Research. 2006;**1110**(1):166-174

[42] Molzhon A. Exploring the influence of socioeconomic status on the executive function and theory of mind skills of preschoolers [dissertation]. Richmond, VA: Virginia Commonwealth University; 2016

[43] Ellis BJ. Toward an adaptation-based approach to resilience. In: The Biology of Early Life Stress. Berlin: Springer; 2018. pp. 31-43

[44] St. John AM, Kibbe M, Tarullo AR. A systematic assessment of socioeconomic status and executive functioning in early childhood. Journal of Experimental Child Psychology. 2019;**178**:352-368

[45] DePrince AP, Weinzierl KM, Combs MD. Executive function performance and trauma exposure in a community sample of children. Child Abuse and Neglect. 2009;**33**(6):353-361

[46] Duncan RJ, McClelland MM, Acock AC. Relations between executive function, behavioral regulation, and achievement: Moderation by family income. Journal of Applied Developmental Psychology. 2017;**49**: 21-30

[47] Liew J, Chen Q, Hughes JN. Child effortful control, teacher–student relationships, and achievement in academically at-risk children: Additive and interactive effects. Early Child Research Quarterly. 2010;**25**(1):51-64

[48] Rhoades BL, Greenberg MT, Domitrovich CE. The contribution of inhibitory control to preschoolers' social–emotional competence. Journal of Applied Developmental Psychology. 2009;**30**(3):310-320

[49] Pears KC, Fisher PA, Bruce J, Kim HK, Yoerger K. Early elementary school adjustment of maltreated children in foster care: The roles of inhibitory control and caregiver involvement. Child Development. 2010;**81**(5):1550-1564

[50] Karbach J, Kray J. How useful is executive control training? Age differences in near and far transfer of task-switching training. Developmental Science. 2009;**12**(6):978-990

[51] Blakey E, Carroll DJ. A short executive function training program improves preschoolers' working memory. Frontiers in Psychology. 2015;**6**:1827

[52] Diamond A, Barnett WS, Thomas J, Munro S. Preschool program improves cognitive control. Science. 2007;**318**(5855):1387-1388

[53] Dowsett SM, Livesey DJ. The development of inhibitory control in preschool children: Effects of "executive skills" training. Developmental Psychobiology: The Journal of the International Society for Developmental Psychobiology. 2000;**36**(2):161-174

[54] Espinet SD, Anderson JE, Zelazo PD. N2 amplitude as a neural marker of executive function in young children: an ERP study of children who switch versus perseverate on the dimensional change card sort. Developmental Cognitive Neuroscience. 2012;**2**:S49-S58

[55] Thorell LB, Lindqvist S, Bergman Nutley S, Bohlin G, Klingberg T. Training and transfer effects of executive functions in preschool children. Developmental Science. 2009;**12**(1):106-113

[56] Viterbori P, Usai MC, Traverso L, De Franchis V. How preschool executive functioning predicts several aspects of math achievement in Grades 1 and 3: A longitudinal study. Journal of Experimental Child Psychology. 2015;**140**:38-55

[57] Kray J, Ferdinand NK. How to improve cognitive control in development during childhood: potentials and limits of cognitive interventions. Child Development Perspectives. 2013;**7**(2):121-125

[58] Traverso L, Viterbori P, Usai MC. Improving executive function in childhood: evaluation of a training intervention for 5-year-old children. Frontiers in Psychology. 2015;**6**:525

[59] Semple RJ, Reid EF, Miller L. Treating anxiety with mindfulness: An open trial of mindfulness training for anxious children. Journal of Cognitive Psychotherapy. 2005;**19**(4):379

[60] Semple RJ, Lee J, Rosa D, Miller LF. A randomized trial of mindfulness-based cognitive therapy for children: Promoting mindful attention to enhance social-emotional resiliency in children. Journal of Child and Family Studies. 2010;**19**(2):218-229

[61] Beveridge M, Jarrold C, Pettit E. An experimental approach to executive fingerprinting in young children. Infant and Child Development: An International Journal of Research and Practice. 2002;**11**(2):107-123

Chapter 2

Musical Training Enhances Inhibitory Control in Adolescence

Claudia L.R. Gonzalez, Frank Robertson and Robbin L. Gibb

Abstract

Music production is a complex activity that involves nearly every function in the brain. Whether skills transfer from musical training to other cognitive abilities is a growing area of research. There is evidence to suggest that musical training in children and adult musicians is associated with an improvement in a variety of executive functions (EFs). This study examined whether those associations are also present during adolescence, and whether there is a relationship between the time spent in musical training and EF. Adolescents between the ages of 14 and 18 completed three tests of EF: Tower of Hanoi to assess working memory, Wisconsin Card Sort Test to assess cognitive flexibility, and Stroop Color Word Task to assess inhibition. They also completed a musical experience questionnaire, including their lifetime musical practice hours. Adolescent musicians were found to have improved inhibitory control (as measured by the Stroop Task) relative to nonmusicians and inhibition correlated with musical practice time. No other elements of EF were found to be associated with musical training. These findings suggest that the impact of musical training may not be the same for all EFs, and that there may be unique associations between this type of training and inhibitory control.

Keywords: executive function, inhibition, music, adolescent, cognitive function

1. Introduction

From lullabies to symphonies, campfires to clubs, birthdays to funerals, music is woven throughout everyday life. Children respond to music starting in their very earliest moments and music is thought to predate speech evolutionarily [1]. Music is a powerful driver of cognitive and neurological development involving the use of nearly every cognitive faculty. Furthermore, it is well known that music engages the appetitive/rewarding neurochemical systems of the brain [2]. The impact of music throughout development is an area of interest across multiple disciplines. Both music and language allow us to communicate through sound, and both require the ability to process and produce precise sounds. The same abilities that allow us to sing and discern emotion from a melody, allows us to discern meaning from words [1]. Music is a highly complex cognitive activity. A musician must coordinate fine motor movements in order to reproduce a memorized series of sounds while receiving auditory, somatosensory, and visual feedback. Becoming an expert musician requires years of dedicated practice. Music has been proposed as an intervention for cognitive and neurological development because of the breadth and depth of the faculties exercised in this activity [3, 4]. It is not just those functions directly recruited to produce music that are impacted by it. Executive functions (EFs) are cognitive abilities that organize and direct the deployment of other cognitive processes and they also benefit from musical training.

EF includes abilities such as working memory, cognitive flexibility, and behavioral inhibition. Working memory is task-oriented memory that allows people to remember what they are doing and to recall relevant information that allows for task completion. Working memory is involved in accomplishing most tests of EF, as participants must at a minimum remember the rules of the task. One task that measures working memory ability is the *Tower of Hanoi* (*ToH*). ToH requires participants to move pieces of a tower across a set of three spaces. The rules of the game are such that this manoeuver takes a minimum of fifteen moves to complete. In order to avoid errors and complete the task in as few moves as possible, participants must keep the rules in mind and think through multiple moves ahead [5]. Working memory is a fundamental EF that allows for the planning and execution of this goal-oriented task. Cognitive flexibility or task switching is an element of EF that requires a person to move back and forth between several tasks successfully. These are the abilities that allow for multitasking. Cognitive flexibility can be measured using a tool like the *Wisconsin Card Sorting Task* (*WCST*) wherein participants complete multiple similar tasks back to back. Researchers measure how seamlessly participants transition to the new task by tracking the errors they make which would have been correct in the previous task [6]. This ability to rapidly switch between tasks is required for successful navigation of a world where many complicated jobs and separate priorities are competing for attention. Inhibition is the ability to resist doing something natural or instinctual and instead engage in some effortful activity. Being able to inhibit a behavior successfully allows one to sort out irrelevant information and remain focused on a given task. Inhibition also allows people to pause and consider other skills that can be used to solve the problems that are important to them. It is no surprise then, that inhibition is critical for academic success. Bull and Scerif [7] studied seven to nine-year olds and discovered that inhibition predicted a child's mathematical ability independent of their intelligence and reading ability. Objective tests of inhibition often ask participants to respond to one type of stimulus while introducing some other competing stimulus that the participant must ignore. A popular test of inhibition is the *Stroop Colour Word Task* (*SCWT*). Here stimuli are presented in pairs and participants are asked to respond to the less salient stimulus. In the classic SCWT, participants are presented with words that denote a color that are printed in different colors (i.e. "green" printed in green ink) and asked to respond to the color of the ink rather than reading the word. When these stimuli are congruent the task is simple, but when they do not match (i.e. "green" printed in red ink) inhibition is required, leading to increased response time and a higher error rate [8].

Better EF is associated with improved outcomes in school and life, and so has been a focus of research in the last decade [9]. Researchers have looked into training EF, particularly inhibition, to improve school performance in children. For example, kindergarten children trained for a month on tasks that promote inhibitory control such as a modified SCWT, achieved a grade one performance level after the training [10]. Another way to enhance inhibitory control and thus academic achievement is through musical training. Short-term musical interventions of a few months to a year have been found to be effective in raising children's EF and verbal intelligence [11, 12, 14]. Children engaged with music have higher intelligence and better inhibitory control than age-matched children without musical training [13–15]. Therefore, inhibitory control interventions are important means to enhance academic performance.

A great deal of research has focused on adult musicians and demonstrates a variety of behavioral and neurological benefits associated with this long-term musical training. Adult musicians show improved EFs compared with nonmusicians in working memory and particularly in inhibitory control [16, 17]. Beyond behavioral research, the brains of long-time musicians have been found to be structurally and functionally distinct from the brains of nonmusicians [18, 19]. These changes are thought to underlie the cognitive benefits found to be associated with musical training.

A gap in the literature is the understanding of how musical training affects cognitive function in adolescence. Adolescence is the period between childhood and adulthood, beginning at the onset of puberty around 11 years of age, and continuing until adulthood [20]. Adolescence is an important period of development; physically, socially, and cognitively. Adolescence and early childhood are both periods of high neuroplasticity and rapid cognitive development. These two windows of elevated neuroplasticity provide opportunities to help youth cultivate the faculties which they will carry with them into adulthood. Because musical training has been so thoroughly demonstrated to enhance cognitive development in early childhood it is worth asking whether musical training in adolescence is also effective in increasing EF skills. Weintraub et al. [21] found evidence for two developmental windows in childhood and adolescence while assessing the cognitive battery included in the NIH Toolbox for the assessment of Neurological and Cognitive Function. They found that in measures of memory, and general EF there was a sharp increase in proficiency between the ages of 3 and 6. A second smaller spike in executive function development occurs starting at 12 years old and continuing until early adulthood at age 25.

The current study investigates the association between musical training and EF in adolescence. Given the previously discussed benefits of musical training on cognitive function in children and adults, we wondered if musical training has the same positive associations with EF development in adolescents? We know that even short musical interventions can have significant impacts on a child's EF, and that child musicians engaged in extracurricular musical training show improved EF across a variety of domains [11, 12]. It is possible that these benefits wash out by the adolescent years, as children without musical training may catch up through other activities. However, if music does have a uniquely strong ability to train EFs as indicated by the existing literature, adolescent musicians will continue to exhibit improved cognitive abilities.

2. Methods

2.1 Participants

Forty adolescents (21 females, 19 males) between the ages of 14–18 were recruited from local middle- and high-schools in Lethbridge Alberta. Participants self-identified as right-handed, and were healthy, with no history of neurological impairment. Participants were not told the purpose of the study, but were told about each of the tasks they would complete before giving consent. Parental consent was obtained for participants younger than 18 before they arrived for testing.

3. Procedure

Each participant completed a music self-report questionnaire, and three tests of EF: the ToH (working memory), WCST (cognitive flexibility), and SCWT (inhibition). The entire experiment took between 35 and 45 min to complete.

3.1 Tower of Hanoi

Four square blocks were stacked on each other, on the first of three marked spaces (see **Figure 1**). Participants began the task centered on the second space, with both hands on the table. They were asked to move the tower of blocks to the third space, stacked in the same order that they began. Participants were only allowed to move one block at a time, and could only stack blocks on top of larger blocks. Participants' hands were filmed while completing this task. Total moves to complete the task were recorded. Completing the task requires a minimum of fifteen moves, and anything lower than twenty is consider good performance.

3.2 Wisconsin Card Sorting Task

This study used a computerized version available on PsyToolkit (https://www.psytoolkit.org/experiment-library/stroop.html) [22]. Four square cards appeared at the top of the screen. Left to right they contained one red circle, two green triangles, three blue crosses, and four yellow stars (see **Figure 2**). A fifth card appeared at the bottom of the screen, containing a random combination of colored shapes. Participants were asked to click the card at the top of the game window that matched the card at the bottom of the game window according to shape, color, or number. Which rule to use was not disclosed to the participant, and changed several times throughout the session. When a participant clicked the correct card, a bell rang and the word "Good" in white flashed on the screen. In the case of an incorrect trial a white "No" flashed on the screen and was spoken by a robotic voice. Total errors were recorded as well as perseveration errors, wherein participants continued using a previous rule (which was formerly correct) in the next round of trials.

3.3 Stroop Color Word Task

This experiment utilized a computerized version of the Stroop available at expfactory.github.io [23]. Participants were instructed to identify the color of words printed on the screen as red, blue, or green, by pressing buttons on the keyboard (**Figure 3**). Each trial began after a 500 ms fixation and words were presented on

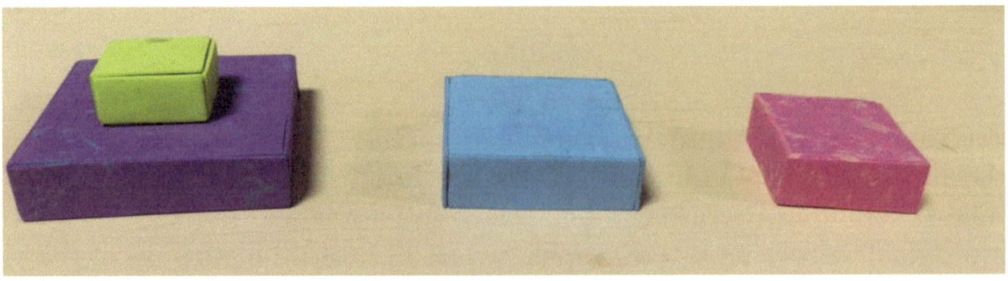

Figure 1.
Tower of Hanoi: this task measures planning and working memory. Participants moved blocks from the left space to the right, according to a set of specific rules. Completing the ToH requires a minimum of 15 moves. Move to complete is the measure of EF in this task.

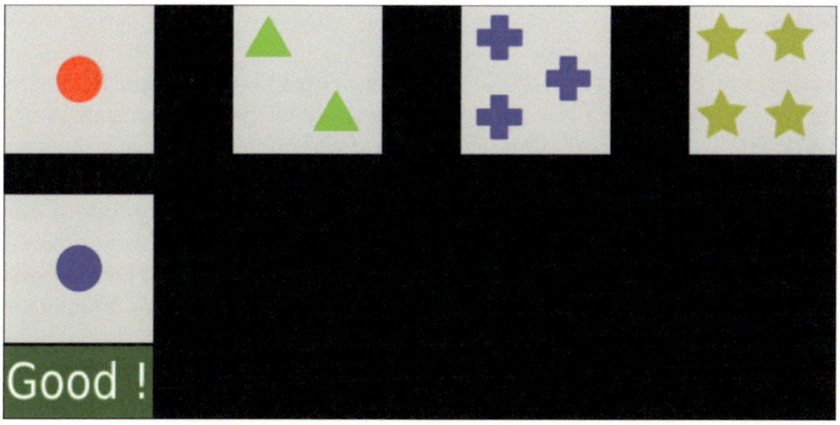

Figure 2.
Wisconsin Card Sort Task: participants clicked on the cards at the top in order to match with the card at the bottom. Cards could match based on the number, color, or type of shapes on the card, and this rule changed throughout the session.

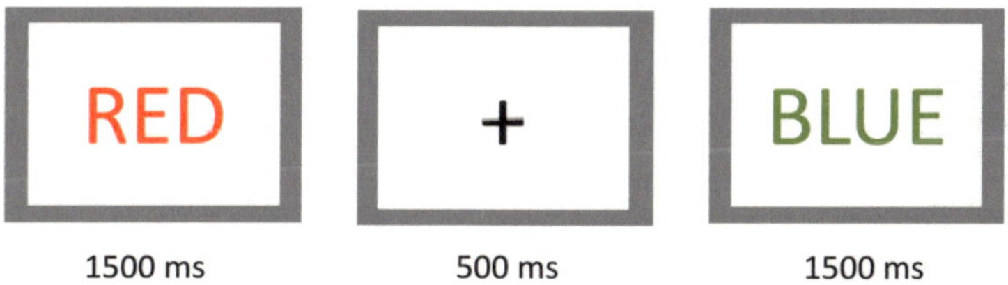

Figure 3.
Stroop Color Word Task: participants responded to a series of words by pressing a key corresponding to the color that the word was printed in. Each word appeared on the screen for 1500 ms. A fixation mark appeared on the screen for 500 ms before each trial. Trials were categorized as congruent and incongruent, and errors were recorded for each condition.

the screen for 1500 ms or until participants responded. Participants completed 23 practice trials, followed by 96 measured trials. Forty-eight of these trials were congruent, meaning the color of the word matched the printed meaning of the word, (e.g. "Red" in red ink). Forty-eight were incongruent, meaning the color of the word did not match its printed meaning, (e.g. "Green" in red ink). Errors were recorded for both the congruent and incongruent conditions (**Figure 3**).

3.4 Music self-report questionnaire

Participants completed a self-report questionnaire detailing their musical training. Each participant reported whether they were currently playing any instruments or singing a vocal part. They reported each of those instruments and gave the time spent practicing each week, and the years spent practicing that instrument. They then repeated the exercise for any musical experience they had in the past and subsequently abandoned. Finally, participants were asked to rank their knowledge of music theory, ability to read music, and general musical aptitude on a five-point Likert scale (1–5), where 1 was no ability and 5 was exceptional.

For the purposes of this study, we considered participants to be musicians if they had at least three years of musical training, and a minimum of five hundred reported lifetime hours engaged in musical training. This eliminated participants who had only just begun engaging with music, and allowed this study to focus on the long-term impacts of musical training.

4. Results

In order to test the hypothesis that teenagers with a history of musical training would have higher executive function than those without, a series of Welch nonparametric T-tests were conducted. This test was chosen because it does not assume normalcy, and is more robust to dependency between multiple comparisons. Musician status was used as the independent variable and number of moves to complete the ToH as well as errors in the WCST and the SCWT were dependent variables. In order to account for multiple comparisons Bonferroni correction was used. SCWT errors were found to be significantly different between musicians and nonmusicians (see **Table 1**). Musicians were found to commit significantly fewer errors than nonmusicians.

Variable	Orientation	Musician mean	Musician SE	Non-musician mean	Non-musician SE	t Statistic	*p*-Value
Tower of Hanoi (moves to complete)	Lower for better EF	32.889	3.53	26.684	3.47	−1.2717	0.5593
WCS errors (preservation errors)	Lower for better EF	7.750	0.770	9.500	1.09	1.2744	0.2124
Stroop errors (total errors)	Lower for better EF	4.389	0.759	9.737	1.40	3.3774	0.0022*

Musicians make significantly fewer errors in the Stroop Task than nonmusicians. Welch Pairwise two tailed T-tests.
**Adjusted for Bonferroni correction.*

Table 1.
Comparison between musicians and nonmusicians on tests of EF.

4.1 Correlation between musical practice time and executive function

In order to examine whether increased musical training time, or self-reported musical ability was associated with executive function, a Pearson's Product-Moment Correlation analysis was performed. This analysis allowed us to treat musicianship as a continuous variable, and to evaluate whether increased musical training time was associated with better EF in the absence of any categories. Musical training time correlated with SCWT Errors; the more musical experience a participant reported, the fewer errors on the SCWT, ($r_{(40)} = -.405; p = 0.01$).

5. Discussion

While music has been demonstrated to have positive associations with EF in childhood and adulthood, the impact that music has on EF throughout adolescence is less well understood. Two research questions were investigated: (1) Does musical training have the same positive associations with EF in adolescence as it does in young children? (2) Is there a relationship between time spent on musical training and adolescent EF? The results of this study showed a positive association of musical training with a key contributor to EF: inhibition. Inhibition, as measured by the SCWT, was the only domain of EF in which adolescents with musical training differed from nonmusicians. Furthermore, the results of the SCWT showed a positive correlation with lifetime musical training (i.e. total number of lifetime practice hours); the more hours engaged in practice, the better the behavioral inhibition in adolescence. Once again, the SCWT was the only measure of EF associated with musical training, indicating that spending more time engaged in musical training results in greater improvements to inhibition. Taken together, these results indicate a unique relationship between musical training and inhibitory control.

During the SCWT participants are asked to parse an incoming stream of information and control their responses in a nonintuitive fashion. This is a central skill set for a musician attempting to properly respond to input from the current sounds, the sheet music, their fellow bandmates, and the sensorimotor feedback that comes with performing a piece of music. Musicians must inhibit a large number of possible responses to these stimuli in order to select the actions that will create the music they wish to produce. Mastering behavioral inhibition to generate the perfect performance is one feature that makes music so rewarding. Imagine a saxophone player attempting to sight read a new melody. The musician reads each oncoming note moments before they have to play it, just like a participant reads the next word in the SCWT as it flashes on the screen. The musician's fingers move to carefully practiced positions, each one unique to the note, just like a participant during the SCWT taps the correct key, unique to the color.

The fact that adolescent musicians in this sample did not show any improvement in the areas of working memory and cognitive flexibility, was somewhat surprising given the results of other studies. A meta-analysis including 18 studies showed improved working memory in children with musical training [24]. Bhide et al. [25] showed that short-term musical training improved working memory in a population of 6 and 7-year-olds who were struggling with reading. The children were engaged in 19 sessions over two months, during which they were given rhythm training. At the end of the two months children were shown to perform significantly better on a digit span backwards test of working memory. Zuk et al. [15] found that working memory and cognitive flexibility was better in both preadolescent children and in adults with musical training. Puzzling, they report that musical training had no influence on inhibitory control in either group. This is in stark contrast to the finding of the present study in which inhibition was found to be most influenced by musical training. Our finding is consistent with other studies in children and adult musicians which have shown that improvement in inhibition is the most reliable effect that musical training has on EF across a variety of tasks, and throughout the lifespan. Children's inhibition improves in response to musical interventions and long-term private music education [3, 12, 14, 15]. Adult musicians have improved inhibition that persists into old age [17, 26, 27]. The current study demonstrates that the relationship between musical training and inhibitory control is not disrupted throughout the tumultuous developmental years of adolescence.

Inhibition may be improved by the dedication required for musical training and thereby lead children to be more effective in developing their cognitive abilities. There is evidence that musical training in children improves inhibition more than other equivalent forms of artistic training. Moreno and colleagues showed that twenty days of musical training was sufficient to improve performance of kindergarten children on a visual Go-No Go task. The children were trained on pitch, tempo, melody, voice, and other basic concepts, using a computer program that focused on listening tasks. These children outperformed an active control group receiving an equivalent fine arts training [3, 12]. This result suggests that there is something especially important about music in the development of inhibition. Furthermore, it appears that musical training is an effective intervention for training inhibitory control. In fact, musical interventions are commonly used to enhance behavior in children with developmental delays, ADHD, and even autism [28, 29].

This form of therapy is also used in people with brain injury and neurodegenerative disorders [30, 31]. Perhaps the common element here is that musical interventions improve inhibitory control which in turn improves behavioral outcomes.

The benefits to inhibition have been shown to persist in adults with a history of musical training. Bialystok and Depage [32] showed that musicians performed better on an auditory Stroop test of inhibition than those with no musical training. This result was confirmed by D'Souza, et al. [27] using a full battery of inhibition tests, including the visual Stroop, a flanker task, and an auditory stop signal test. Musicians showed a significant advantage on each of these measurements compared with adult nonmusicians. These improvements continue even as people age. In a study of professional musicians older than age 50 [26], musicians were found to outperform nonmusicians in a full battery of inhibition tasks. This battery included an auditory Stroop task, a go-no-go task, a distracted reading task and a Simon task (in which a color appeared on one side of the screen, and participants had to hit a matching button which was on the same side as the color in congruent trials and on the opposite side in incongruent trials). Music practice can thus be beneficial throughout life.

It is possible that certain kinds of musical practice improve inhibition better than others. Bialystok and Depage [32] did not find any difference between vocalists and instrumentalists in their study, however recent findings have suggested that there may be differences between different kinds of musical training. For example, percussionists who must keep careful track of time may have better inhibition than other musicians. A study compared inhibition abilities between vocalists, percussionists, and nonmusicians between the ages of 18 and 35 [33]. The authors found that percussionists outperformed both vocalists and nonmusicians in inhibitory control. This finding further supports the notion that musical training which involves more inhibitory control improves this EF.

5.1 Limitations and future research

The current study has a number of limitations. A relatively small sample size meant that subdivisions between different types of musicians were inappropriate. This study only accepted participants in mid and late adolescence, making developmental inferences more difficult. The correlational nature of this study makes it impossible to make determinations about cause and effect. Finally, the uncertainty about the relationship between various EF's, and overlap in how these functions are measured is a general problem in this field which this study did not address. Future research could be designed in such a way that tackles these issues and allows for a more thorough understanding of adolescent EF.

Few studies have explicitly examined distinctions between forms of musical training, and this should be a priority for future research investigating relationships between musical training and cognitive abilities. A study directly examining the differences between vocalists and percussionists in EF found that percussionists out-performed vocalists, and nonmusicians in the area of inhibition [33]. Previous research has shown no difference in inhibition between vocalists and instrumentalists, which only serves to make the enhanced abilities of percussionists even more interesting [32]. The timing of musical training is another factor which might lead to distinct outcomes. Early musical training has been shown to increase the volume of the corpus callosum in the brain whereas later training does not [34]. An implication of this finding is that musical training will have a larger effect if it occurs within early development. These findings indicate that some subdivisions by age of musical training and by musical speciality may be important to the EF differences observed here. This study was unable to account for these potential distinctions due to the limited sample size.

Extra-curricular musical training means practicing for hours every week. While other children may take a break, or not have an opportunity to engage in a cognitive exercise after school, music students are translating dots on a page into music in the air. This extra period of instruction and practice may itself be the cause of the improved cognition observed across the board in musicians. It is also true that musical instruction costs money. This means that the average musician may be of higher socioeconomic status, which could be a potential confound when interpreting the current results. Intervention studies, where music lessons can be provided regardless of economic status, and musical training that can be compared against equally challenging programs are needed to address these issues.

While this study does establish a relationship between inhibition and musical training in adolescents, it is unclear whether musical involvement in the adolescent years is truly responsible for this improvement. It is possible that childhood musical training contributes in important ways to the effect observed here. Similarly, it is possible that adolescents with stronger inhibitory skills are more likely to continue engaging in musical training even as they gain more independence in the mid adolescent years. In order to address this issue, it would be necessary to give adolescents musical interventions in the style that has been used to improve childhood EF.

6. Conclusion

The current study examined the relationship between musical training and EF in mid to late adolescence. Musical training was found to be associated with better inhibition, as measured by the SCWT but not working memory or cognitive flexibility. Future research should focus on determining causality, and accessing whether it is feasible to use music to improve inhibitory control in adolescents.

Author details

Claudia L.R. Gonzalez[1,2*], Frank Robertson[1,2] and Robbin L. Gibb[1,2]

1 The Brain in Action Laboratory, Department of Kinesiology, University of Lethbridge, Canada

2 Department of Neuroscience, Canadian Centre for Behavioural Neuroscience, University of Lethbridge, Canada

*Address all correspondence to: claudia.gonzalez@uleth.ca

References

[1] Levman BG. The genesis of music and language. Ethnomusicology. 1992;**36**:147-170

[2] Chanda ML, Levitin DJ. The neurochemistry of music. Trends in Cognitive Sciences. 2013;**17**:179-193

[3] Moreno S, Bidelman GM. Examining neural plasticity and cognitive benefit through the unique lens of musical training. Hearing Research. 2014;**308**:84-97

[4] Zatorre R. Music, the food of neuroscience? Nature. 2005; **434**(7031):312

[5] Humes GE, Welsh MC, Retzlaff P, Cookson N. Towers of Hanoi and London: Reliability and validity of two executive function tasks. Assessment. 1997;**4**:249-257

[6] Berg EA. A simple objective technique for measuring flexibility in thinking. Journal of Experimental Psychology. 1948;**39**:15-22

[7] Bull R, Scerif G. Executive functioning as a predictor of children's mathematics ability: Inhibition, switching, and working memory. Developmental Neuropsychology. 2001;**19**:273-293

[8] MacLeod CM. Half a century of research on the Stroop effect: An integrative review. Psychological Bulletin. 1991;**109**:163-203

[9] Diamond A, Lee K. Interventions shown to aid executive function development in children 4-12 years old. Science. 2011;**333**:959-964

[10] Zhang Q, Wang C, Zhao Q, Yang L, Buschkuehl M, Jeggi SM. The malleability of executive function in early childhood: Effects of schooling and targeted training. Developmental Science. 2019;**22**:e12748

[11] Janus M, Lee Y, Moreno S, Bialystok E. Effects of short-term music and second-language training on executive control. Journal of experimental child psychology. 2016;**144**:84-97

[12] Moreno S, Bialystok E, Barac R, Schellenberg EG, Cepeda NJ, Chau T. Short-term music training enhances verbal intelligence and EF. Psychological Science. 2011;**22**(11):1425-1433

[13] Hennessy SL, Sachs ME, Ilari B, Habibi A. Effects of music training on inhibitory control and associated neural networks in school age children: A longitudinal study. Frontiers in Neuroscience. 2019;**13**:1080

[14] Schellenberg EG. Long-term positive associations between music lessons and IQ. Journal of Educational Psychology. 2006;**98**(2):457

[15] Zuk J, Benjamin C, Kenyon A, Gaab N. Behavioral and neural correlates of EFing in musicians and non-musicians. PLoS One. 2014;**9**(6):e99868

[16] Degé F, Kubicek C, Schwarzer G. Music lessons and intelligence: A relation mediated by EFs. Music Perception: An Interdisciplinary Journal. 2011;**29**(2):195-201

[17] Moussard A, Bermudez P, Alain C, Tays W, Moreno S. Life-long music practice and executive control in older adults: An event-related potential study. Brain Research. 2016;**1642**:146-153

[18] Gaser C, Schlaug G. Brain structures differ between musicians and non-musicians. Journal of Neuroscience. 2003;**23**(27):9240-9245

[19] Schneider P, Scherg M, Dosch HG, Specht HJ, Gutschalk A,

Rupp A. Morphology of Heschl's gyrus reflects enhanced activation in the auditory cortex of musicians. Nature Neuroscience. 2002;**5**(7):688

[20] Blakemore SJ, Choudhury S. Development of the adolescent brain: Implications for executive function and social cognition. Journal of Child Psychology and Psychiatry. 2006;**47**:296-312

[21] Weintraub S, Dikmen SS, Heaton RK, Tulsky DS, Zelazo PD, Bauer PJ, et al. Cognition assessment using the NIH Toolbox. Neurology. 2013;**80**(11 Suppl 3):S54-S64

[22] Psytoolkit. Available from: https://www.psytoolkit.org/experiment-library/stroop.html

[23] Burleigh T, Sochat V. Web-based Stroop Task. 2018. Available from: https://osf.io/9pc46/

[24] Sala G, Gobet F. When the music's over. Does music skill transfer to children's and young adolescents' cognitive and academic skills? A meta-analysis. Educational Research Review. 2017;**20**:55-67

[25] Bhide A, Power A, Goswami U. A rhythmical musical intervention for poor readers: A comparison of efficacy with a letter-based intervention. Mind, Brain and Education. 2013;**7**:113-123

[26] Amer T, Kalender B, Hasher L, Trehub SE, Wong Y. Do older professional musicians have cognitive advantages? PLoS One. 2013;**8**(8):e71630

[27] D'Souza AA, Moradzadeh L, Wiseheart M. Musical training, bilingualism, and EF: Working memory and inhibitory control. Cognitive Research: Principles and Implications. 2018;**3**(1):11. DOI: 10.1186/s41235-018-0095-6

[28] Antonietti A, Colombo B, DeRocher BR. Music Interventions for Neurodevelopmental Disorders. Cham: Palgrave Pivot; 2018

[29] Wan CY, Schlaug G. Neural pathways for language in autism: The potential for music based treatments. Future Neurology. 2010;**5**:797-805

[30] Leggieri M, Thaut MH, Fornazzari L, Schweizer TA, Barfett J, Munoz DG, et al. Music intervention approaches for Alzheimer's disease: A review of the literature. Frontiers in Neuroscience. 2019;**13**:132

[31] Vik BMD, Skeie GO, Specht K. Neuroplastic effects in patients with traumatic brain injury after music-supported therapy. Frontiers in Human Neuroscience. 2019;**13**:177

[32] Bialystok E, DePage AM. Musical expertise, bilingualism, and EFing. Journal of Experimental Psychology: Human Perception and Performance. 2009;**35**(2):565

[33] Slater J, Azem A, Nicol T, Swedenborg B, Kraus N. Variations on the theme of musical expertise: Cognitive and sensory processing in percussionists, vocalists and non-musicians. European Journal of Neuroscience. 2017;**45**(7):952-963

[34] Steele CJ, Bailey JA, Zatorre RJ, Penhune VB. Early musical training and white-matter plasticity in the corpus callosum: Evidence for a sensitive period. Journal of Neuroscience. 2013;**33**(3):1282-1290

Chapter 3

Addiction: Brain and Cognitive Stimulation for Better Cognitive Control and Far Beyond

Xavier Noël, Antoine Bechara, Mélanie Saeremans, Charles Kornreich, Clémence Dousset, Salvatore Campanella, Armand Chatard, Nemat Jaafari and Macha Dubuson

Abstract

Addiction behaviors are characterized by conditioned responses responsible for craving and automatic actions as well as disturbances within the supervisory network, one of the key elements of which is the inhibition of prepotent response. Interventions such as brain stimulation and cognitive training targeting this imbalanced system can potentially be a positive adjunct to treatment as usual. The relevance of several invasive and noninvasive brain stimulation techniques in the context of addiction as well as several cognitive training protocols is reviewed. By reducing cue-induced craving and modifying the pattern of action, memory associations, and attention biases, these interventions produced significant but still limited clinical effects. A new refined definition of response inhibition, including automatic inhibition of response and a more consistent approach to cue exposure capitalizing on the phase of reconsolidation of pre-activated emotional memories, all associated with brain and cognitive stimulation, opens new avenues for clinical research.

Keywords: addiction, inhibition, brain stimulation, memory reconsolidation, cue exposure

1. Introduction

Despite considerable progress in detoxification, pharmacology, and psychological interventions in addictive behaviors, clinical outcomes remain suboptimal (e.g., high relapse rate or poor quality of life) [1]. The main reason of the poor clinical outcomes is likely to be related to multiple interacting determinants of social, psychological, and biological mechanisms involved in the addiction risk and the relapse, a view that is not compatible with pure essentialism and simplistic approaches of addiction [2].

Inter-individual variations within the addiction group in respect to neurobiological mechanisms of addiction were highlighted by influential theorizations [3–9]. Indeed, addictive behaviors can be viewed as the product of an imbalance between separate, but interacting, neural systems: an impulsive, largely amygdala-striatum-dependent, neural system that promotes automatic, habitual, and salient behaviors; a reflective, mainly prefrontal cortex-dependent, neural system for decision-making, forecasting the future consequences of a behavior, and inhibitory control; and the insula that integrates interoception states into conscious feelings and decision-making processes that are involved in uncertain risk and reward. Any imbalance in the dynamics of these systems can account for poor decision-making (i.e., prioritizing short-term consequences of a decisional option), and the lack of willpower [10–12], which heightens the risk for addiction and relapse.

As part of the "executive network" involving ventrolateral prefrontal cortex and dorsolateral prefrontal cortex, response inhibition interacts with automatic behavioral ("habit network") and motivational responses ("reward network") to produce flexible actions and adaptive choices. Indeed, the inhibition of a prepotent response has become an important element of the responsible braking system and limiting the expression of spontaneous motivation and emotion signals [13]. Indeed, successful self-regulation requires the ability to inhibit impulses that are not compatible with one's goals [14].

Importantly, psychostimulant dependence, alcohol dependence, and gambling disorders have been consistently associated with a response inhibition deficit [5]. However, the deficit in inhibition observed in addiction population is generally of low or moderate effect size [15, 16]. Nevertheless, even a small effect size can have clinically relevant effects, as evidenced by the impact of impaired response inhibition on the risk of dependence and response to treatment [9, 17–19]. Indeed, response inhibition is considered as a primary candidate for cognitive remediation that can potentially reduce the risk of addiction and the relapse [20]. As an alternative way consistent with dual-process theories, to limit these risks is to reduce the need for inhibitory control, for instance, by dampening automatic conditioned responses (e.g., craving, attentional and memory biases) triggered by contextual (e.g., the sight of a bottle of beer) or internal (e.g., negative effects) cues. In addition, more automatic forms of response inhibition could be trained in the hope of enabling individuals to generate appropriate alcohol-stop associations without too much of an effortful process [21].

In this chapter, we investigate the manner the risk associated with too limited response inhibition can be reduced by implementing multiple forms of cognitive training, invasive and noninvasive brain stimulation techniques, and neurofeedback (NF). It should be noted that an overwhelming majority of neuroscientists engaged in brain stimulation in psychopathology has truly viewed brain-based interventions as complementary interventions to clinical treatments such as cognitive-behavioral therapy and motivational enhancement intervention [22, 23]. Indeed, the beliefs, desires, emotions, and intentions of patients are essential elements to take into account [2], which can be modulated by brain- and cognitive-based interventions.

After a brief presentation of response inhibition theories and methods, we summarize cognitive training intervention in the context of addictive behaviors as well as three brain stimulation techniques (i.e., deep brain stimulation, electric and magnetic brain stimulation) and finally protocols of neurofeedback. We then develop more complex clinical and research concepts (e.g., combined cognitive training and brain stimulation along with cue exposure interventions).

2. Executive functioning, response inhibition, and self-regulation: terminological and theoretical clarifications

Numerous terms have often been used to describe similar concepts. For example, concepts such as self-regulation, inhibition, executive function, cognitive control, effortful processes, impulsivity, risk-taking, and disinhibition are sometimes clearly delineated but sometimes are used as synonyms or closely related concepts [24]. Attempts to clarify those concepts (e.g., the degree that some of those constructs overlap) have been scarce but mostly suggest that intrinsic aspects of regulation, self-regulation, serve as an umbrella concept that encompasses top-down and bottom-up processes that mutually influence one another [24–26]. Naturally, the influence of extrinsic aspects of regulation, that is, facilitated or hindered self-regulation due to others' mind and action, is far to be negligible and should be considered to fully apprehend the determinants of dysregulated actions, such as addictive behaviors [27, 28].

2.1 Inhibition in definition

As suggested by William James, "Voluntary action, then, is at all times a resultant of the compounding of our impulsions with our inhibitions" [29]. In order to control the desire, the reason takes place as represented like Plato seeing the will as a charioteer attempting to control two horses (one of desire and one of reason) in Phaedrus. For both Hippocrates and Aristotle, the body and mind are not independent, but each influences the other. Long after, the fundamental duality between reason and emotion conferred to will the essence to control (or inhibit) action and emotion. A few decades later, Sherrington was awarded the 1932 Nobel Prize for Physiology and Medicine for his contribution to our understanding of inhibition in neurophysiology, which consolidated the concept.

Although creating a sense of comfort in theorizing, the explanation (e.g., brain structure in the frog that inhibits a spinal reflex) based on similarity to excitatory or inhibitory functions of the nervous system (i.e., neurons can serve either functions) that strong impulses can be impeded through the implementation of inhibition remains a debated matter [30].

Because of this warning, presenting an operational definition of "inhibition" remains an adventurous venture, not only because of the weight of its intuitive load (e.g., cognitive inhibition is equivalent to neural inhibition sometimes as metaphor) but also because of the phenomenon and explanation conflation or a confusion between a causal process and a functional relationship [31].

In most cases, response inhibition mainly refers to the suppression of actions that are no longer required or that are inappropriate, which supports flexible and goal-directed behavior in ever-changing environments [32]. As such, given its role in supervising ongoing thoughts and action in working memory, response inhibition has been considered as a hallmark of executive functions [33, 34]. As a form of top-down (intentional) inhibition process, prepotent response inhibition refers to deliberate inhibition operating on basic and reactive elements of action, which is essentially non-automatic and represents a cost. Intentional control depends on motivation and capacity [35]; it is subjectively deliberate, slow, and sequential; and it requires working memory and is capacity-limited.

However, a growing amount of data challenged this strictly hierarchical view [36, 37]. Indeed, executive control emerges from an interactive and competitive network generating biases in advance and is strongly influenced by personal recent and past experiences. Indeed, humans automatize as much as possible; hence apparent intentional inhibition can in fact operate automatically for particular contexts, due to context-inhibition associations made through learning. For instance, on the stop-signal task [32], when people are informed that they may have to stop a response in the near future, they typically slow down operation through altering activity in lower-level systems that are involved in stimulus detection, action selection, and action execution [38]. Put differently, instead of relying only on executive functioning, low-level and high-level systems work together for self-regulation.

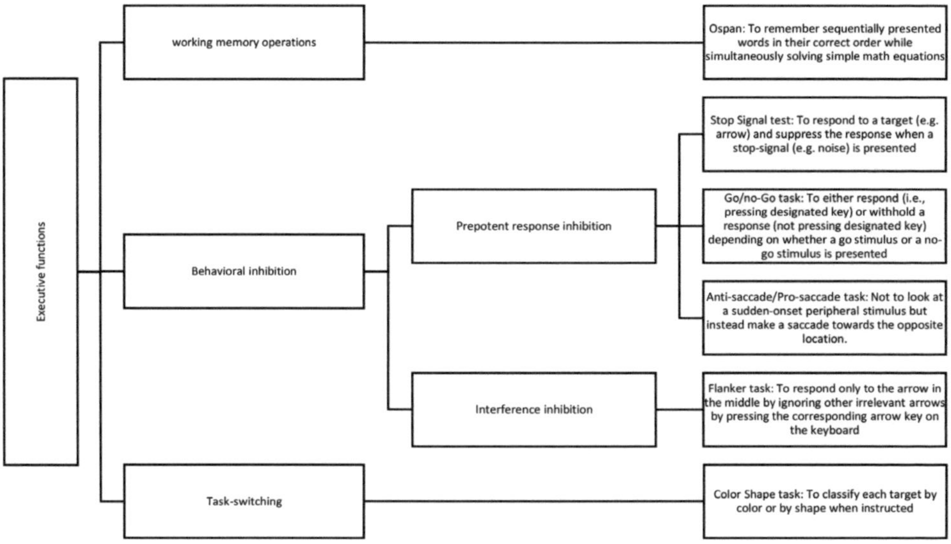

Figure 1.
Executive function classification proposed by [33].

Although closely related to executive functioning, response inhibition can be distinct from other forms of executive functions such as working memory update (i.e., the ability to replace information stored in working memory with new information) and switching (i.e., the ability to shift attention to other tasks or perceptual dimensions) [33] (see **Figure 1**).

Based on latent variable analysis, several forms of response inhibition could be distinguished [39–42]. A first distinction has been made between the inhibition of prepotent response and the resistance to distracter interference. However, the robustness of this two-factor solution remains questionable in light of low correlations between inhibition measures, when the contribution of memory processes was intentionally reduced [41]. It follows from this discussion that studies using a single laboratory paradigm for assessing or investigating inhibition do not warrant generalization beyond the specific paradigm studied.

More fine-grained forms of inhibition have been put forward across the years [39, 41]. Indeed, resistance to proactive interference consists of resisting memory intrusions from information that was previously relevant to the task but has since become irrelevant.

A second categorization relies on the degree of anticipation and preparation of response inhibition [43, 44]. Reactive inhibition (or reflexive inhibition) is a form of inhibition that one can implement without anticipation (e.g., stopping the car when an animal unexpectedly jumps on to the road). Proactive inhibition refers to the impact of inhibition preparation on the inhibitory performance (e.g., keeping one's foot close to the brake after passing a warning sign for animals on the road). Possibly because proactive form of response inhibition requires much more than just inhibition, as attested by shared brain contribution of both forms of inhibition (the right inferior frontal gyrus, supplementary motor area and striatum) and also specific engagement of working memory-related regions (i.e., dorsolateral prefrontal region) [45], proactive inhibition may be more ecologically valid than reactive inhibition [46].

Sufficient agreement can be found on the contributions of these different inhibitory control mechanisms as measured by a variety of cognitive tasks described by Friedman and Miyake [39]. The list of tasks includes the color Stroop, anti-saccade, stop-signal, simon, global-local, and negative compatibility tasks that could share a component of inhibition of prepotent response; the letter flanker, the number Stroop, arrow flanker, and negative compatibility as well as the task assessing n-2 repetition costs tend to assess resistance to distracter interference.

3. Response inhibition and addiction

Consistent with the previous discussion, response disinhibition is an important element of modern addiction models [6, 9], and empirical data support this claim, particularly for gambling, psychostimulant, and alcohol addiction [5]. By conferring a central position to response inhibition, brain imaging and behavioral studies demonstrated abnormal functioning in individuals at risk to develop an addictive behavior, in addicted people, and in individuals who relapsed [9, 47, 48]. Indeed, a variety of response inhibition deficits are present in numerous forms of reinforcement pathologies (e.g., tobacco dependence [49, 50], alcohol disorder [51, 52], eating disorders [53, 54], gambling disorder [55] (but see [56])). Second, those deficits can predict relapse in drug and behavioral addiction [18, 57, 58], and research suggests that recently abstinent addicts experience heightened difficulties with response inhibition [59, 60]. Thirdly, the inability to stop one's actions, due notably to early stressful life events and negative parent–child interaction [61], can influence behavioral and substance addictions later in life [17, 61].

In addition, it should be noted that impaired response inhibition has a strong impact in important aspects of decision-making. For instance, impaired prepotent response inhibition in alcoholics was associated with poorer performance on the Iowa gambling task [62], which requires participants to deal with uncertainty in a context of punishment and reward, with some choices being advantageous in the short term (high reward) but disadvantageous in the long run (higher punishment) and known for its ecological validity of decision-making [63–65]. Risk-taking could also be modulated through inhibitory control engagement, with participants being more cautious once anticipating to suppress their response [66]. Unfortunately, the benefit of this form of inhibitory training is fragile and transitory [67]. Besides, data from a sample of pathological gamblers revealed no effect of this procedure on risk-taking [68]. Finally, prepotent response inhibition can moderate the behavioral expression of implicit cognition [69]. Indeed, the impact of implicit cognitive processes on drinking behavior should be stronger in individuals with relatively weaker executive control than in individuals with relatively good executive control, as shown by using the classical Stroop interference scores [70]. Conversely, among adolescents with relatively good executive control, explicit expectancies were the best predictor of alcohol use [71].

In theory, prepotent response inhibition can directly be involved in *myopic* decision, that is, a preference for dominant sooner-smaller at the detriment of less salient larger-later decisions [72]. Steeper delay discounting rate is indubitable in individuals with addiction [73], which concurs to the risk of addiction and treatment response [74, 75]. In support of the existence of a relationship between prepotent response inhibition and short-termism, decreased gray matter volume in lateral prefrontal regions is associated with greater impatience [72, 76]. However, the level of inhibitory control, as typified by the stop-signal reaction time of the stop-signal task [32], and preference for large delayed rewards, as assessed using delay-discounting paradigms, are generally *not* correlated in both healthy participants [77] and clinical populations (e.g., in patients with attention deficit/and hyperactivity disorder) [78], which suggests that response inhibition and delay discounting are independent factors, each of them contributing to addiction.

4. Cognitive training

As mentioned earlier, several findings argued in favor of cognitive-based interventions aimed at targeting response inhibition as an assistant in preventing relapse in addicted population.

Amending those deficits is a huge endeavor and ways to achieve it is still a debated matter [79]. This section elaborates on several cognitive training interventions (CTI) that potentially impact positively on inhibition-related processes in individuals with reinforcement pathologies.

4.1 Restoring inhibitory control

Two contrasting approaches have been used to evaluate response inhibition training on substance use disorders and behavioral addiction: general stop inhibition with classical paradigms assessing prepotent response inhibition or with versions adapted to the type of addictive behaviors (e.g., *alcohol* Stroop test or *cocaine* go/no-go task).

Although there is no conclusive evidence of true increase in inhibitory control in response to extensive training with standard go/no-go or SST tasks in adults [80], training of inhibitory control reduced monetary risk-taking [66] and alcohol-seeking [81]; even this effect is small and short-lived [67, 68], which could potentially explain why some studies failed to observe far-transfer effects [82].

In contrast to some studies using formal training of working memory (e.g., [83]) to evaluate their direct impact on unhealthy behaviors (e.g., alcohol abuse), which can be positive in nonclinical samples [84], but not clinical population [85], modified versions of response inhibition tasks have served as training paradigms [79, 86–90].

During "inhibitory control training" (ICT), participants complete an inhibitory control task (go/no-go task, stop-signal task, anti-saccade task) in which the requirement to exercise inhibitory control is paired with cues related to healthy behaviors, before the effects of this training on the target behavior are measured (for reviews, see [79, 89, 91]). For example, when a group of participants in whom inhibition was paired with neutral cues was compared, participants who completed a stop-signal task in which alcohol images were paired with inhibition subsequently led to reduced ad libitum alcohol consumption in the laboratory, but not self-reported drinking in the week after training [90]. In the same vein, participants who learned to associate food images with inhibition on a go/no-go task subsequently consumed less of those foods when given access to them [88]. In contrast, training of oculomotor inhibition in the presence of alcohol-related cues led to slowed eye movements toward target cues on catch trials, but this manipulation failed to influence the proportion of inhibitory failures and had no influence on alcohol consumption in the laboratory [90]. Initial results indicated that the relationship between behavioral inhibition and alcohol intake may be causal, possibly to the ecological value of alcohol motor response inhibition paradigms (e.g., picking up a glass of alcohol beverage may be directly targeted by motor inhibition training), and training of oculomotor inhibitory control is far less convincing.

Meta-analytic approach [89, 91, 92] demonstrated that the effect of ICT on behavior was dependent on the task used. In theory, research on inhibition have led to the recognition that there are at least two types of inhibitory control: action restraint in which the decision to inhibit is made from the onset (go/no-go tasks) and action cancelation in which the decision to inhibit occurs after implementation of the prepotent response (stop-signal task) [93, 94]. However, the meta-analyses reveal that the higher the proportion of successful inhibitions of appetitive signals, the greater the magnitude of the effect of ICTs. Indeed, studies found a larger and more statistically robust ICT effect size when go/no-go rather than stop-signal tasks are used. One reason for the superiority of training action restrain on action cancelation [95, 96] is that compared to go/no-go tasks, stop-signal tasks have a lower rate of overall stop success that ends up hindering the development of strong stimulus-stop associations [53, 95]. Instead, go/no-go tasks feature strong stimulus-stop association due to the rate of successful inhibitions reflected in the number and proportion of stop-stimulus pairings, which in turn moderate the effects of training on unhealthy behavior. It is still in debate to ascertain what repeated stop-stimulus pairings could cause: better intentional inhibitory control over impulsive action [97], facilitated automatic retrieval of stimulus-stop associations [21, 37, 98], or diminished motivational properties of target information [99–101]. The issue of which mechanisms mediate the relationship between cognitive training paradigms and behavioral changes remains highly complex for several reasons. First, the size of behavioral change is at best rather small and does not survive more than a couple of hours [67]. Besides, it remains to be seen whether the control condition used in most of the studies where participants are required to rapidly respond to appetitive stimuli as often as inhibiting responses contributes to inflated effect size of ICT [89]. Second, there is no clear consensus on theoretical constructs such as motivation, where generally there is a weak relationship between implicit and explicit measures of stimulus evaluation [102]. Indeed, whereas a majority of studies using implicit motivational measures demonstrate no effect of inhibition of cognitive training on stimulus devaluation, other studies using Likert scale or other explicit procedures [101] demonstrated devaluation effects following this sort of intervention [103–105].

To sum up, general or cue-specific inhibition training has yielded only modest clinical results, and mechanisms remain to be elucidated.

4.2 Cognitive bias modification

Cognitive bias modification consists of pairing alcohol-related content with action tendencies, classically pushing a joystick in response the alcohol-related images and pulling the same joystick in response to soft drinks [106, 107]. Cognitive and clinical effects of this procedure have been compared to sham training conditions requiring an equal number of approach and avoidance movements to both alcohol and soft drinks pictures (i.e., no stimulus-response contingency). Main original outcomes are (a) reduced alcohol approach-related biases indicated with the implicit association task and (b) reduced alcohol relapse up to 1 year after the training. As suggested, an important mediating effect was the building of an alcohol-avoidance bias [106]. The clinical efficacy of this approach regardless of patients' characteristics (age, number of prior detoxifications, etc.) has shown to be too limited to be integrated as such in clinical settings. Indeed, on a meta-analysis of 14 studies (mainly for alcohol and tobacco use problems) involving 2435 participants [22], the authors found a small, nonsignificant overall effect on cognitive bias assessed directly after the completion of the training intervention. In addition, neither smoking nor alcohol reduction was found in response to training intervention. In the same vein, a recent meta-analysis "cast serious doubts on the clinical utility of CBM interventions for addiction" [108]. In response to this assertion, influential researchers in the field, Wiers et al., argued that this analysis combined the results of laboratory and randomized controlled trials, which may underestimate CBM's actual effectiveness when incorporated into regular therapy [109].

In addition to those theoretical and methodological limitations, several moderators could hinder yet existing ICT effects. It is the case of the degree of readiness to change, that is, the goal to gain control over harmful behaviors that make the ICT intervention more congruent with the participant's mindset, hence potentiating its effects [110]. Another source of variation in the effect of ICT could be the strength of appetitive responses to food cues [111], with the effects of ICT on behavior being proportional to the strength of appetitive responses to cues before ICT [112, 113]. Whether individual differences in attempts to limit drinking, smoking, or gambling moderate the effects of ICT on alcohol intake is a promising avenue for future research. Put together with current literature revealing substance-specific relapse (and vulnerability)-related impairments, it is recommended to investigate cognitive training programs based on a patient-tailored protocol [114].

5. Brain neurostimulation techniques

5.1 Brain stimulations: noninvasive and invasive techniques

Effects of brain stimulation of basic processes, neurochemical regulation, and cognitive and affective processes at the system level have revealed promising results when applied to addiction treatment (for reviews and meta-analyses, see [23, 115, 116]). The most used stimulation techniques include deep brain stimulation, repetitive transcranial magnetic stimulation, and transcranial direct current stimulation known for their effect on self-regulatory processes and possibly acting on several forms of response inhibition.

5.2 Invasive brain stimulations

5.2.1 Deep brain stimulation

Despite ethical concerns due to potential serious side effects [117], deep brain stimulation has expanded from successful thalamic stimulation for Parkinsonian tremor (for a review, see [118]) to psychiatric conditions including addiction [23, 115, 116]. DBS is a neurosurgical procedure involving the placement of a neurostimulator, often called "brain pacemaker," which delivers electrical impulses through implanted electrodes to specific brain regions related to abnormal functioning characterizing neurological and psychiatric conditions.

Back in the 1980s, BDS was introduced as treatment for movement disorders and became well known for treating the tremor of patients with Parkinson disease [119]. During the 2000s, it started to be applied in psychiatric disorders when the pathology is treatment-refractory: in obsessive-compulsive disorder (OCD) [120] and in major depression [121]. DBD gained interest as a means to treat addiction as soon as studies reported unintended alleviation of comorbid alcohol [115], nicotine [122], and gambling [123] addictions.

As reviewed by Luigjes et al. [124], based on a total of eight studies, bilateral high-frequency NAc stimulation in heroine dependence came with reduced craving and prolonged abstinence. In addition, animal studies have provided evidence that NAc DBS dampens impulsivity [125, 126], which represents a core aspect of addictive behaviors [127].

However, because of the absence of double-blind controlled trials in addiction, the cost and the invasiveness of the procedure, as well as the lack of consensus regarding its clinical efficacy and the encountered difficulties to recruit motivated participants [128], DBS to treat addiction could suffer from feasibility issues.

5.3 Noninvasive brain stimulations

Because they offer a safe economical way to modulate brain activity, techniques such as repetitive transcranial magnetic stimulation and transcranial direct current stimulation are growing in popularity for interventions in psychiatric disorder [129, 130]. They are so-called noninvasive to reflect the fact that the magnetic pulses are delivered from a coil placed over the scalp, without a surgical intervention (in contrast to DBS), which contributed to its popularity as techniques for modulating brain activity over the past two decades. Although recent reviews repeatedly recommended more clinical trials before firm conclusions about their efficacy could be drawn [124], their effects on key addictive-related phenomena (e.g., craving, impulsivity) are noteworthy [131].

5.3.1 Repetitive transcranial magnetic stimulation

Repetitive transcranial magnetic stimulation delivers in a time interval a magnetic pulse through the skull via a stimulating coil. The magnetic field involves a focal electrical current, depolarizing underlying cortical neurons. The intensity, duration, properties, localization, and frequency directly influence the effects. Low frequency (1–5 Hz) tends to produce inhibitory effects and fits well the intention of downregulating activity in the targeted regions [132, 133]. High frequency (10–20 Hz) tends to produce excitatory effects on the stimulated brain area. However, substantial inter-individual responses to both low- and high-frequency stimulation have been reported [134]. By using either figure-of-eight coils or H-coils known to produce highly focal stimulation in superficial cortex or deeper intracranial penetration to a more central target, respectively [135], the clinical influence of a variety of clinical phenomena has been investigated.

rTMS and addictive behaviors: The most frequently used rTMS setup has been 10 sessions of stimulation on either the right DLPFC with a high frequency or the left DLPFC with lower frequency. In nicotine addiction, frequently reported findings include reduced transitory (no longer than several weeks following the intervention) cue-induced craving for cigarette as well as lower nicotine consumption [136, 137]. Interestingly, an important placebo effect has been repeatedly found in rTMS studies. Indeed, a reduction in the daily consumption of alcohol [138] or cocaine [139] has been found in response to both active and sham stimulation. In the same vein, although a reduced attentional bias toward alcohol cues has been found in response to high-frequency left DLPFC rTMS, all participants (irrespective of their stimulation condition) reported a reduced craving [140]. The placebo response should be due to a concurrent treatment regimen, which too often is missing from these studies, and better study designs should involve participant blinding.

Regarding the clinical impact of rTMS in behavioral addiction (e.g., gambling addiction, binge eating), the insufficient number of controlled trials prevents drawing conclusion [23].

An important issue to be discussed is the potential cognitive mediators of rTMS effects in addicted subjects. In theory, a reduction in craving intensity and in substance use could be mediated by improved response inhibition or mental flexibility or a change in salience or automatization. No effects above sham stimulation were found on prepotent response inhibition evaluated by a go/no-go task [141].

Although DLPFC is critical for cognitive-executive functions, stimulation of medial regions tends to influence affective-motivational functions [142]. This region along with others such as the insula is important for the selection of long-term over short-term reward, an interplay that may be abnormal in individuals with addictive behaviors [143, 144]. Magnetic stimulation of the medial prefrontal cortex may bias the preference for delayed, over sooner, rewards [145]. However, this encouraging view has been recently tempered by a study reporting the absence of effect of rTMS targeting the medial prefrontal cortex on impulsive choice on the delay discounting task in pathological gamblers [146].

In contrast to rTMS that requires 20–30 min of stimulation time to achieve its full effect, theta burst stimulation (TBS) protocols could achieve similar efficiency by employing protocols lasting between 20 s and 3 min that induce NMDA receptor-dependent long-term potentiation and long-term depression [147]. A recent meta-analytic review [148] that focused on healthy participants on the prefrontal cortex with theoretically linked cognitive test performance as the outcome revealed that uninterrupted train of TBS decreases performances on measures of inhibitory control, attentional control, and working memory, whereas intermittent TBS has positive effects on executive functions (but not likely ceiling effects). Future studies comparing different magnetic stimulation protocols should be conducted in the context of addictive behaviors.

5.3.2 Transcranial direct current stimulation

Transcranial direct current stimulation involves delivering low-intensity electric current (typically 0.5–2 mA) via electrodes placed on the scalp and/or upper body. Cortical excitability is modulated by a polarity-dependent shift of the neuronal membrane potential [149, 150]. On the macroscopic level, anodal stimulation enhances cortical excitability via depolarization and long-term potentiation, whereas cathodal stimulation inhibits excitability via hyperpolarization and long-term depression [149]. The density, duration, and direction of the current that comes into contact with underlying neurons determine the strength and direction of neuromodulation [149, 150]. After an initial subthreshold depolarization or hyperpolarization of neuronal membrane potentials that increases or decreases the likelihood of spontaneous neural firing, facilitation of long-term potentials or long-term depression occurs [151]. tDCS modulation of the action potentials even lasts beyond the stimulation period [149, 150], and several neuromodulation sessions could increase the duration of the effects [152].

tDCS as an intervention in addictive disorders: a recent review [23] showed that seven published studies have focused on the impact of tDCS on various measures related to substance addiction. Despite important inter-individual differences in response to tDCS [153], most preeminent effects were found on craving reduction [154]. In addition, mixed results were found with respect to executive control functions [124, 131, 155, 156]. Importantly, in healthy controls no improvement was found after tDCS stimulation of bilateral DLPFC stimulation of either right anodal/left cathodal or left anodal/right cathodal on decision-making under risk (e.g., balloon analogue task), an absence of effect possibly due to a ceiling effect [157].

The benefit from reducing cue-induced craving for clinical population could be pertinent. Indeed, pressing, urgent, and irrepressible desire to drink or to smoke has been strongly associated with *loss of control*, leading to a high relapse rate [158]. However, the mediating effect of craving variation in response to tDCS on relapse is not obvious. For instance, in a tDCS study in patients with alcohol dependence (two daily stimulations 5 consecutive days on left cathodal/right anodal over the dorsolateral prefrontal cortex), no differences with regard to changes on scores of craving were found despite an improved overall perception of quality of life and reduced relapse probability in several alcoholics [159]. In nicotine addiction, right anodal stimulation on the DLPFC reduces craving with minimal heterogeneity, whereas cathodal tDCS on this region showed the most positive effect on cue-provoked craving and smoking intake [154]. However, this craving reduction, which may be due to increased control on cue reactivity, could be too small to positively impact cigarette use. Indeed, as compared to sham, active tDCS significantly reduced smoking craving and increased brain reactivity to smoking cues within the right posterior cingulate, as measured with a functional magnetic resonance imaging event-related paradigm, but failed to diminish the number of cigarettes smoked (see also [160]) and the exhaled carbon monoxide 1 month following the stimulation [161].

Regarding the association between tDCS and food, reduction of food craving [162–164] and calorie intake [97] in healthy subjects and reduced craving for food in overweight subjects [165] have been reported.

Mediating processes involved in brain stimulation of the PFC is likely to be more complex than previously expected. It was demonstrated that anodal tDCS applied over frontoparietal regions has previously been shown to enhance attention and executive control functions [166–168], but the effects are limited and non-lasting.

Working memory, depending on the stimulation modalities, can be a valid candidate mediator [169]. As a multicomponent system responsible for temporary storage and manipulation of information, working memory sustained emotional regulation [14]. Because many psychiatric disorders are associated with working memory impairments, it may be useful to improve the transient "online" manipulation of emotional thoughts in treatment rehabilitation.

Response inhibition is another good candidate mediator of the relationship between tDCS and clinical change. For instance, a recent study showed that tDCS over the right inferior frontal cortex made healthy participants more efficient in proactive, but not reactive, inhibition [170]. In another study, tDCS over the pre SMA during a stop-signal task increases activity in the pre SMA after anodal stimulation during stop trials and was associated with improved inhibitory control [171]. Finally, after applying tDCS over the rIFG, two studies [170, 172] observed a decrease in P3 amplitude during no-go and/or stop trials in anodal compared to inactive stimulation. The clinical value of those results in the case of addictive behaviors remains to be seen. One possibility is that a reduction of P3 amplitude during successful response inhibition on a go/no-go task in response to tDCS could be a protective factor for the risk of relapse in vulnerable alcoholics, that is, those with greater amplitude of P3 [173].

The clinical impact of tDCS on substance use can be still more subtle. For instance, in obese participants, electric brain stimulation on the DLPFC facilitated the transition between unconscious and conscious perception of appetitive stimuli, a phenomenon particularly pronounced in participants with higher body mass index [174]. Those findings could have an impact on craving regulation, via augmented awareness of implicit determinants of craving, enhancing the risk of relapse.

Although the proposed cognitive mediators presented in this section showed promising results, their clinical relevance is still tentative. Much more data is needed to achieve a better comprehension of the impact of tDCS on addictive behaviors.

5.3.3 Neurofeedback

In neurofeedback, participants learn to modulate their own brain activity through feedback. The main goal is for participants to develop effective self-regulation strategies to increase desired brain activity. Functional magnetic resonance imaging neurofeedback (fMRI-NF) and electroencephalography neurofeedback (EEG-NF) are the most developed configurations [175], each with its strengths and weaknesses [176, 177]. Higher spatial resolution and broad brain coverage characterize fMRI-NF [178], while EEG-NF has very good timing but low spatial accuracy. In EEG-NF, it is possible to modify neuronal oscillations in specific frequency domains associated with functions such as attention or relaxation. fMRI-NF and its variant, real-time fMRI [179], provide direct feedback to modulate (increase or decrease) neuronal activity in the regions of interest [180]. With fMRI-NF, brain regions of interest are defined a priori on the basis of consensual articles describing which neurocognitive networks are altered and predictive of low use of controlled substances [181]. In EEG-NF, critical oscillations in certain frequency bands have been associated with mental states (e.g., alpha and theta frequencies for a relaxed or meditative state, beta rhythm, or sensorimotor for inhibition).

In the context of addictive behaviors, alpha-theta and the alpha-theta augmented with SMR training represent the two main protocols of EEG-NF. As pointed out by [23], only a few studies have reached a reasonable quality (only one study used a control condition matched in time) [182], which makes it difficult to determine which protocol provides the best results. However, in two studies [182, 183], a reduction in the number of false alarms (i.e., response to no-go trials) on a go/no-go task was observed in participants who received EEG-NF rather than an alternative treatment. It is interesting to note that sensorimotor interferences can be reduced in healthy participants who undergo SMR neurofeedback training, which they have learned to voluntarily increase, resulting in better cognitive performance [184].

With respect to fMRI-NF, an analysis based on eight studies [23] revealed that six of them performed on nicotine addiction showed better regulation at the level of the anterior part of the cingulate gyrus directly associated with a decrease in the desire to smoke [185]. In alcohol addiction, reduced craving was achieved by modifying activity in the ACC, PFC, and insula [186]. Further studies should explore reward (e.g., ventral striatum) and control processing before the clinical relevance in addiction could be confirmed and mediating factors (e.g., prepotent response inhibition) identified.

6. A step forward: combined interventions with retrieval-extinction techniques

Coupling brain stimulation with other pharmacological and non-pharmacological interventions may provide further knowledge about individual brain oscillation states across several montages and voltages as well as long-term structural and functional effects of brain stimulation on addicted patients [187]. These proposals will certainly make better use of brain stimulation techniques and therefore optimize their clinical effects (**Table 1**).

Here we focused more on the effects of combined interventions to improve clinical efficacy. Combined methodologies have provided positive clinical results in a variety of psychiatric conditions [188]. From a broad perspective, the use of neuromodulation techniques to promote brain plasticity [189, 190] while exerting response inhibition, extinction learning, or cognitive restructuration may help regain control over prepotent actions.

As shown in **Table 2**, only five studies used several combined approaches in the context of substance use disorders. The results are rather disappointing. Indeed, in five out of five studies, no interaction between brain stimulation and cognitive manipulation was found, indicating that tDCS did not add any clinical value to behavioral training. However, two studies have examined the combined effects of left anodal tDCS on DLPFC and cognitive-behavioral modification (CBM) in high-risk drinkers undergoing or not treatment. In the high-risk drinker sample, 1.0 mA was administered on left DLPFC during three CBM sessions for 3 to 4 days. No effect of CBM or tDCS was observed on approach bias or alcohol consumption. However, participants reported a reduced craving during a signal responsiveness task [191]. In treatment seekers, 2.0 mA over left DLPFC over the course of four

Brain stimulation and investigation techniques	
Deep brain stimulation (DBS)	A small device, similar to a pacemaker, is surgically implanted to deliver electrical stimulation to targeted areas of the brain
Transcranial direct current stimulation (tDCS) and its variant, the transcranial alternating current or random noise stimulation	Allows changes in cortical activity to be generated by inducing a direct low-intensity (1–2 mA) current in the brain
Repetitive transcranial magnetic stimulation (rTMS)	Induces repeated single magnetic pulses in the brain to modulate cortical activity
Event-related potentials (ERP)	By means of electrodes placed at various points on the scalp and amplified through an EEG machine, the ERP measures electrical potentials generated by the brain in response to specific internal or external events (e.g., sensory, cognitive, or motor stimuli)
Function magnetic resonance imagery (fMRI)	To detect regional and time-varying changes in brain metabolism and blood oxygenation
Cognitive training and related cognitive functions	
Domain-general cognitive training	A structured practice of mental abilities that are used to solve complex tasks regardless of their content (e.g., working memory)
Domain-specific cognitive training	A structured practice of mental abilities where the semantic content of the processed information is controlled (e.g., negative emotional words or alcohol-related content)
Cognitive biases	These refer generally to unidentified or inaccurately identified attitudes or stereotypes, but in the present essay, we reported attentional, memory, and action tendency biases as normal and abnormal manifestations of domain-specific processing (e.g., attentional engagement toward smoking cues in deprived smokers)
Cognitive deficits	Describes a deviation from the normal functioning of general cognitive domains (e.g., episodic memory, executive functioning)
Executive functions	Partially independent, top-down processes reflecting goal cognitive corresponding to an internal goal are involved in the control of behavior, emotions, and cognition. The updating of the relevant information, the inhibition of prepotent impulses, and the mental set shifting are core functions
Proactive control	Refers to expectancy-based activation of cognitive control (maintaining goal activation to bias responding) prior to an anticipated conflict or challenge. In contrast, reactive control refers to the activation of cognitive control after a change or conflict is detected
Working memory	The ability to hold multiple things in mind at once while mentally manipulating one or more of them (e.g., updating)
Interference control	Ignoring (inhibiting, suppressing, or deactivating) internal or external competing information to protect working memory or to focus attention on goal-relevant information
Prepotent inhibition response	Refers to the suppression of actions that are no longer required or that are inappropriate, which supports flexible and goal-directed behavior in ever-changing environments
Self-regulation	Encompasses cognitive control, emotion regulation, and top-down and bottom-up processes that alter emotion, behavior, or cognition to attempt to enhance adaptation (or to achieve an explicit or implicit goal or goal state)
Learning-related concepts	
Conditioned stimulus	A previously neutral stimulus that has been learned to predict an outcome; the presentation of the stimulus evokes the memory of the previous learning

Extinction	The presentation of a conditioned/learned stimulus now in the absence of the previously associated outcome; this results in the temporary decline of subsequent memory expression
Learning	The behavioral changes of an organism are the result of regularities in the environment of that organism
Reactivation	Re-exposure to memory reminders, which may result in destabilization of the previously learned neural representation of memory
Retrieval	A reminder results in recollection of the previously learned memory; the term encompasses the multiple processes from reactivation of the neural memory representation to behavioral expression of the memory
Reconsolidation	The active process that is necessary to restabilize a reactivated/destabilized memory; disruption of reconsolidation results in memory impairment, while new information is incorporated during reconsolidation into an updated memory
Reactivation-extinction (retrieval-extinction)	The combination of memory reactivation (usually via a reminder that results in memory retrieval) and, after a brief interval, subsequent extinction

Table 1.
Definitions and glossary of major terms as relevant in the current essay.

training sessions in 4 consecutive days was used [192]. No significant interaction effect for the full sample was found. However, in this study, there were some indications of a boosting effect of tDCS and CBM, such that relapse was lower in this group at the 1-year follow-up.

More encouraging evidence for the usefulness of a combined approach comes from research on patients with mood disorders. For instance, participants with social anxiety disorder had a significant decrease in attention bias for threatening signals during single anodal stimulation as opposed to simulated stimulation [196]. In obsessive-compulsive disorder, exposure to information aimed at generating a conditioned response (e.g., increase anxiety in response to a risk of contamination) has been tested in combination with tDCS [197] or rTMS [198]. Indeed, by using a personalized provocation of symptoms aimed at generating an appropriate level of distress, the goal was to activate the corresponding neural circuit. During brain stimulation, people were asked to think about provocation ("Please keep thinking about your dirty hands"). Positive results were found in this combined setting (brief exposure therapy + tDCS or rTMS). In the field of nicotine addiction, one study has shown that it is advantageous to use a challenge with actual exposure to tobacco signals just prior to the rTMS high-frequency stimulation treatment [199]. It should be noted that this approach requires that the interventions be individualized according to the conditioned responses involved in the addictive process.

Brain stimulation techniques could also be advantageously coupled with interventions targeting the learning process of extinction in addictive disorder. Extinction refers to the disappearance of a conditioned behavior in the absence of positive or negative reinforcement [200]. Extinction is the basis for an intervention based on exposure, a primary treatment for a variety of psychiatric conditions, including addiction [201]. Unfortunately, the extinguishing procedures did not simply wipe out the conditioned responses of the past, as shown by the return of the targeted behavior by extinction which is again apparent after the passage of time, after the presentation of the unconditioned stimulus, and when extinguished signals are encountered outside the extinction context [201]. Instead, extinction may be a new form of learning that exists with extinction memories in distinct neural

Studies	Condition	Inclusion criteria	Exclusion criteria	N	Mean age (SD)	Female/ male	Design	Experimental condition	Outcome measures	Results
den Uyl et al. [191]	Electrophysiological and behavioral effects of combined tDCS and Alcohol Approach Bias Retraining (AABR) in hazardous drinkers	Heavy drinkers want to reduce drinking Dutch-speaking 18–35 years AUDIT > 8	tDCS criteria*	78	21.8 (3.2)	51/27	2 × 2 factorial design: • Active tDCS during active training • Sham tDCS during active training • Active tDCS during sham training • Sham tDCS during sham training	Three sessions of AABR** while receiving tDCS over DLPFC (1 mA for 15 min; 35 cm^2 anode F3 and 100 cm^2 cathode over contralateral supraorbital region)	Alcohol use, craving, AAT, IAT, EEG P300 Quantity of alcohol use at month follow-up	No effects on EEG and behavioral measures of repeated CBM and/or tDCS, except for an effect of tDCS on induced craving
den Uyl et al. [191]	A clinical trial with combined tDCS and Alcohol Approach Bias Retraining in alcohol-dependent patients	Individuals with AUD under a 3-month hospital treatment	tDCS criteria*	91	47 (8.8)	30/91	Three groups in parallel design: • Active tDCS during active training • Sham tDCS during active training • Active tDCS separate from active training	Four sessions of AABR** while receiving tDCS over DLPFC (20 min, 2 mA; 35 cm^2 anode F3 and 100 m^2 cathode F4)	3-month, 1-year abstinence follow-ups, craving intensity, approach bias	No effect of repeated CBM and/or tDCS on 3 months of abstinence duration, craving, and alcohol biases, except a trend-level effect of active tDCS during active training on relapse rate at 1 year only when comparing to sham tDCS (p = .07)

Studies	Condition	Inclusion criteria	Exclusion criteria	N	Mean age (SD)	Female/ male	Design	Experimental condition	Outcome measures	Results
den Uyl et al. [193]	Clinical trial with combined tDCS and Attentional Bias Modification (ABM) in alcohol-dependent patients	Individuals with AUD under a 3-month hospital treatment	tDCS criteria*	83	48.6 (0.9)	21/62	2 × 2 factorial design: • Active tDCS during active ABM • Sham tDCS during active ABM • Active tDCS during sham ABM • Sham tDCS during sham training	Four sessions of ABM*** combined with tDCS (20 min, 2 mA, over DLPFC, 35 cm^2 anode F3, and 100 m^2 cathode F4)	1-year abstinence follow-up, alcohol bias, craving intensity	Stronger avoidance bias only during training session in active tDCS with active ABM ($p < 0.05$) No effects of tDCS and ABM on the bias scores, craving, or relapse
Sedgmond et al. [194]	Effect of tDCS on food consumption or food craving when combined with inhibitory control training in healthy subjects	Healthy participants	In diet to lose weight History of eating disorders Previously participated in this type of study	172	20.81 (0.26)	141/172	2 × 2 factorial design: • Active tDCS during active training • Sham tDCS during active training • Active tDCS during sham training • Sham tDCS during sham training	One session of ICT**** while receiving tDCS over DLPFC (2 mA for 20 min; 35 cm^2 anode F4 and cathode F3)	Food craving, snack buffet consumption, inhibitory control	No evidence for the effect of tDCS on food consumption or food craving with Bayesian. No effect of tDCS on inhibitory control

Studies	Condition	Inclusion criteria	Exclusion criteria	N	Mean age (SD)	Female/ male	Design	Experimental condition	Outcome measures	Results
Claus et al. [195]	Effect of combining CBM and tDCS on reduction of alcohol approach biases and alcohol consumption	At-risk alcohol drinkers AUDIT > 8	History of treatment for AUD or desire for treatment Alcohol withdrawal Brain injury Psychotropic medications Pregnancy Illicit drug use Metal in the body	79	24.5 (2.7)	Not indicated	2 × 2 factorial design: • Active tDCS during active training • Sham tDCS during active training • Active tDCS during sham training • Sham tDCS during sham training	Four sessions (of 1 h per week, 4 consecutive weeks) of AABR** while tDCS right inferior frontal gyrus (2 mA; 20 min; 11 cm^2 anode F10 and the cathode arm)	Drinks per drinking day (DDD) and percent heavy drinking days (PHDD) at baseline, the follow-up visits at 1-week and 1-month follow-ups, alcohol approach bias at baseline	Significant alcohol approach biases at baseline; neither CBM, tDCS, nor the interaction reduced the bias at the follow-up No significant effect of intervention on either DDD or PHDD

tDCS criteria: epilepsy, multiple sclerosis or other neurological illness, previous brain injury/infection, metal in the brain, pacemaker, pregnancy, claustrophobia, recent fainting/panic attack, frequent headaches or dizziness, and eczema or other skin conditions
**Alcohol Approach Bias Retraining: pull or push alcohol or soft drink pictures with joystick.*
***Attentional Bias Modification: dot-probe training task with alcohol, nonalcohol, or object pictures*
****Inhibitory control training: a go/no-go training task with fatty food, healthy food, and close pictures*

Table 2.
Effect of tDCS and behavioral interventions combined in substance use disorder.

circuits [202]. Therefore, increased extinction with new approaches has been extensively studied in animals and, more recently, in humans with aversive responses (e.g., fear) and appetite disorders (e.g., addiction) [203]. The extinction of the conditioned response may be more effective if it is preceded by a brief exposure to the conditioned response, that is to say, a phase of reactivation of the memory [204–206]. This approach, often named *super-extinction*, gave rise to theories of synaptic consolidation [207], which brought a fresh look at memory processes involved in flexible actions. Briefly, once activated, conditioned responses are rendered labile and unstable that interfering intervention (e.g., propranolol administration [208], non-pharmacological manipulation [209, 210]) ensuing during the reconsolidation window could update original memory traces [204]. Reduced involvement of the inhibitory networks [211] and induced plasticity [209] during extinction following reactivation could represent some of the key mechanisms in play. Importantly, whereas in extinction amygdala's representation remains intact, the prefrontal activated reconsolidation would eliminate the necessity of such inhibition [211]. Additionally, as shown in animal studies, one factor that may initiate memory destabilization and reconsolidation is the detention of prediction errors (*surprise effect*) [212, 213]. In humans, some procedures combining prediction errors and memory reconsolidation interference have yielded interesting results in subjects with high alcohol consumption ([214, 215], p. 20; [216]). Although the clinical impact of those essays was not overwhelming, subtle changes of alcohol attractiveness have already been highlighted, such as a reduction of craving for alcohol [216] and significant reductions in verbal fluency for positive alcohol-related words [215]. In theory, conditioned stimuli could be erased with a single treatment, which could solve the compliance problems necessary to continue treatment, promoting abstinence [217]. Although promising and extremely relevant in the context of the prevention and treatment of addictive behaviors, the precise recovery conditions required to successfully destabilize memory remain unclear (e.g., role of prediction error, type of intervention post-activation, counter-conditioning, interference, extinction).

We suggest here that the *super-extinction* procedure can be implemented in combination with brain stimulation techniques and cognitive response inhibition training, for example, which may lead to stronger and more prolonged clinical effects in drug and behavioral addictions. Indeed, not only is the activation of relevant brain circuitry important before the application of brain stimulation [197–199], but it is also possible to capitalize on the lability of memory during reconsolidation. Indeed, reactivated memory becomes labile after retrieval through a process known as memory reconsolidation. Memory reconsolidation after retrieval may be used to maintain or update long-term memories, reinforcing or integrating new information into them [204–206, 209], a phenomenon that would underlie change in psychotherapy [218]. Interestingly, decreasing DLPFC activity has been observed in repeated encounters with memories (e.g., [115]), resulting in a stabilization of memory. Consistently, the stimulation of the control network via an anodal TDCS applied to the right DLPFC during repeated access to acquired information disrupts the long-term retention of these memories [219]. Based on these findings, it is likely that stimulating the control network during reconsolidation of emotional memories associated with addictive behaviors could result in disrupted storage, particularly in circumstances that generate interferences (e.g., training *alcohol-stop* associations). Future research is needed to test these hypotheses and shed new light on this theoretical reasoning.

Another promising possibility is that cognitive training works better when combined with other forms of clinical intervention aimed at enhancing motivation, self-esteem, family functioning, social support, etc. [220]. In other words, a very interesting line of research is to study the interaction between the mechanisms involved in clinical interventions that lead to positive outcomes and the aforementioned cognitive interventions. Too often, clinical interventions have been described simply as a set of technical tools (e.g., CBT, family therapy) instead of mechanisms and processes of clinical interventions (e.g., compensatory skills, self-understanding) [221], which is a problem when we consider that each participant does not respond in the same way to a given intervention. For this reason, it may be that only the participants who benefit most in some way from a given clinical intervention are those for whom cognitive training and brain stimulation work best. It is obvious that the weakness of this hypothesis is precisely the problem encountered by research in identifying central mechanisms and methods related to psychological change in response to clinical interventions [222].

Finally, some studies have found that addicted participants have preserved automatic inhibitory resources [52]. In this study, recently detoxified alcoholics and healthy participants performed a modified stop-signal task that consisted of a training phase in which a subset of the stimuli was consistently associated with stopping or going and a test phase in which this mapping was reversed. In the training phase, stop performance improved for the consistent stop stimuli, compared with control stimuli that were not associated with going or stopping. In the test phase, go performance tended to be impaired for old stop stimuli. Combined, these findings support the automatic inhibition hypothesis. Importantly, performance was similar in both groups, which indicates that automatic inhibitory control develops normally in individuals with alcoholism. Furthermore, clinical interventions aimed at potentiating the automatic suppression of alcohol-going associations combined with procedures encouraging the automatic selection of alternative responses (e.g., intention implementation [223]). This approach has the merit to promote better inhibitory control of the action without saturating the resources of effortful self-regulation. Whether intensive addiction cues/stop associations could benefit from reactivation of craving or negative emotions is an important hypothesis to be tested in further experiments.

7. Concluding remarks

Many efforts have been made to modify the acquired motivational properties of addiction cues and to reinforce the control of prepotent responses via cognitive training, brain stimulation, and neurofeedback protocols. To date, our review has highlighted some of the promises as well as the obstacles that we need to overcome. In keeping with recent narrative critiques and the meta-analytic approach, the current state of the art appears to be like a half-empty or half-full glass. On the one side, an important limitation is the absence of a robust consensus about methods and mechanisms of brain stimulation techniques (but see for a recent consensus, article [224]) and recent findings calling into question inhibition as a psychometric construct [41]. The main consequence of this is the high level of variation between subjects in response to brain stimulation as well as a poor understanding of the precise cognitive mechanisms that mediate the efficacy of brain stimulation. On the other side, the glass could be considered half-filled because a reduction in the state of cue-induced craving is now feasible and the ongoing research on possible moderators could add important information. Indeed, the motivation for change of participants that refers to personal goals and values is a clinical target requiring specific psychological interventions before cognitive and brain enhancement can turn into robust clinical effects [109]. Clearly, the brain (e.g., using EEG or fMRI) and cognitive (e.g., impaired executive functions, exacerbated approach tendencies toward addiction cues) profiles of patients sensitive to cognitive improvement are important factors to identify [114, 225].

In this chapter, we also strongly recommend that conditioned stimuli and conditioned responses that lead to the loss and recovery of control of addictive behavior be better identified and used with retrieval-extinction techniques in combination with brain and cognitive stimulations. If ethical questions arise when unpleasant sensations are felt by people seeking care and when an intervention alters the substance of a memory, as it may disrupt a sense of self, we must remember the lack of effectiveness of contemporary clinical and experimental treatments in an intolerable situation which we have become too accustomed. We hope to have convinced the reader that in reconsolidation-based treatments, even if boundary conditions begin to be discovered [226, 227], the potential benefits may far outweigh the risks.

It is difficult to obtain better cognitive control, such as improving executive functions in adults, as shown by considerable data [80], but capitalizing on preserved automatic inhibitory resources could prove useful for promoting better inhibitory control of the action without saturating the resources of effortful self-regulation [21, 52].

In sum, these are exciting days where a number of key elements useful to change addictive behaviors have now been identified, yet their perfect fit remains to be done. What is also promising is the undeniable need to bridge the gap between experimental studies and clinical issues in taking into account motivation, relevant personal conditioned responses, acute and chronic stress, memory, response inhibition, and brain and cognitive stimulation to provide addicts with better control of their impulse and obsessions because it is often a prerequisite to return to a satisfactory quality of life.

Author details

Xavier Noël[1*], Antoine Bechara[2], Mélanie Saeremans[1], Charles Kornreich[1], Clémence Dousset[1], Salvatore Campanella[1], Armand Chatard[3], Nemat Jaafari[4] and Macha Dubuson[1]

1 Psychological Medicine Laboratory, Faculty of Medicine, Université Libre de Bruxelles, Belgium

2 Department of Psychology, Southern California University, USA

3 Faculty of Psychology, University of Poitiers, France

4 Faculty of Medicine, University of Poitiers, France

*Address all correspondence to: xnoel@ulb.ac.be

References

[1] Miller PM, Book SW, Stewart SH. Medical treatment of alcohol dependence: A systematic review. International Journal of Psychiatry in Medicine. 2011;**42**(3):227-266

[2] Borsboom D, Cramer A, Kalis A. Brain disorders? Not really... why network structures block reductionism in psychopathology research. The Behavioral and Brain Sciences. 2018;**24**:1-54

[3] Goldstein RZ, Volkow ND. Drug addiction and its underlying neurobiological basis: Neuroimaging evidence for the involvement of the frontal cortex. The American Journal of Psychiatry. 2002;**159**(10):1642-1652

[4] Goldstein RZ, Volkow ND. Dysfunction of the prefrontal cortex in addiction: Neuroimaging findings and clinical implications. Nature Reviews. Neuroscience. 2011;**12**(11):652-669

[5] Lee RSC, Hoppenbrouwers S, Franken I. A systematic meta-review of impulsivity and compulsivity in addictive behaviors. Neuropsychology Review. 2019;**29**(1):14-26

[6] Noël X, Brevers D, Bechara A. A neurocognitive approach to understanding the neurobiology of addiction. Current Opinion in Neurobiology. 2013;**23**(4):632-638

[7] Redish AD, Jensen S, Johnson A. A unified framework for addiction: Vulnerabilities in the decision process. The Behavioral and Brain Sciences. 2008;**31**(4):415-437 discussion 437-487

[8] Tang Y-Y, Posner MI, Rothbart MK, Volkow ND. Circuitry of self-control and its role in reducing addiction. Trends in Cognitive Sciences. 2015;**19**(8):439-444

[9] Zilverstand A, Huang AS, Alia-Klein N, Goldstein RZ. Neuroimaging impaired response inhibition and salience attribution in human drug addiction: A systematic review. Neuron. 2018;**98**(5):886-903

[10] Bechara A, Noel X, Crone EA. Loss of willpower: Abnormal neural mechanisms of impulse control and decision making in addiction. In: Handbook of Implicit Cognition and Addiction. Thousand Oaks, California: Sage publications, Inc., 2006. pp. 215-232

[11] Noël X, Bechara A, Brevers D, Verbanck P, Campanella S. Alcoholism and the loss of willpower: A neurocognitive perspective. Journal of Psychophysiology. 2010;**24**(4):240-248

[12] Noël X, Van Der Linden M, Bechara A. The neurocognitive mechanisms of decision-making, impulse control, and loss of willpower to resist drugs. Psychiatry (Edgmont (Pa.: Township)). 2006;**3**(5):30-41

[13] Evans JSBT. Dual-processing accounts of reasoning, judgment, and social cognition. Annual Review of Psychology. 2008;**59**:255-278

[14] Hofmann W, Schmeichel BJ, Baddeley AD. Executive functions and self-regulation. Trends in Cognitive Sciences. 2012;**16**(3):174-180

[15] Argyriou E, Davison CB, Lee TTC. Response inhibition and internet gaming disorder: A meta-analysis. Addictive Behaviors. 2017;**71**:54-60

[16] Lipszyc J, Schachar R. Inhibitory control and psychopathology: A meta-analysis of studies using the stop signal task. Journal of the International Neuropsychological Society: JINS. 2010;**16**(6):1064-1076

[17] Nigg JT, Wong MM, Martel MM, Jester JM, Puttler LI, Glass JM, et al.

Poor response inhibition as a predictor of problem drinking and illicit drug use in adolescents at risk for alcoholism and other substance use disorders. Journal of the American Academy of Child and Adolescent Psychiatry. 2006;**45**(4):468-475

[18] Noël X, Sferrazza R, Van Der Linden M, Paternot J, Verhas M, Hanak C, et al. Contribution of frontal cerebral blood flow measured by (99m)Tc-Bicisate spect and executive function deficits to predicting treatment outcome in alcohol-dependent patients. Alcohol and Alcoholism. 2002;**37**(4):347-354

[19] Whelan R, Watts R, Orr CA, Althoff RR, Artiges E, Banaschewski T, et al. Neuropsychosocial profiles of current and future adolescent alcohol misusers. Nature. 2014;**512**(7513):185-189

[20] Noël X, Brevers D, Bechara A. A triadic neurocognitive approach to addiction for clinical interventions. Frontiers in Psychiatry. 2013;**4**:179

[21] Verbruggen F, Best M, Bowditch WA, Stevens T, McLaren IPL. The inhibitory control reflex. Neuropsychologia. 2014;**65**:263-278

[22] Boffo M, Zerhouni O, Gronau QF, van Beek RJJ, Nikolaou K, Marsman M, et al. Cognitive bias modification for behavior change in alcohol and smoking addiction: Bayesian meta-analysis of individual participant data. Neuropsychology Review. 2019;**29**(1):52-78

[23] Luigjes J, Segrave R, de Joode N, Figee M, Denys D. Efficacy of invasive and non-invasive brain modulation interventions for addiction. Neuropsychology Review. 2019;**29**(1):116-138

[24] Nigg JT. Annual research review: On the relations among self-regulation, self-control, executive functioning, effortful control, cognitive control, impulsivity, risk-taking, and inhibition for developmental psychopathology. Journal of Child Psychology and Psychiatry, and Allied Disciplines. 2017;**58**(4):361-383

[25] Diamond A. Executive functions. Annual Review of Psychology. 2013;**64**:135-168

[26] Zhou Q, Chen SH, Main A. Commonalities and differences in the research on Children's effortful control and executive function: A call for an integrated model of self-regulation. Child Development Perspectives. 2012;**6**(2):112-121

[27] Fals-Stewart W, O'Farrell TJ, Hooley JM. Relapse among married or cohabiting substance-abusing patients: The role of perceived criticism. Behavior Therapy. 2001;**32**(4):787-801

[28] Sripada CS, Angstadt M, McNamara P, King AC, Phan KL. Effects of alcohol on brain responses to social signals of threat in humans. NeuroImage. 2011;**55**(1):371-380

[29] James W. Talks to Teachers on Psychology: And to Students on Some of Life's Ideals. New York: H. Holt; 1899

[30] MacLeod C, Dodd M, Sheard E, Wilson D, Bibi U. In opposition to inhibition. In: The Psychology of Learning and Motivation. Vol. 43. San Diego, CA: B.H. Ross; 2003. pp. 163-214

[31] Smith R. Inhibition: History and Meaning in the Sciences of Mind and Brain. Berkeley: University of California Press; 1992

[32] Logan GD, Cowan WB, Davis KA. On the ability to inhibit simple and choice reaction time responses: A model and a method. Journal of Experimental

Psychology. Human Perception and Performance. 1984;**10**(2):276-291

[33] Miyake A, Friedman NP, Emerson MJ, Witzki AH, Howerter A, Wager TD. The unity and diversity of executive functions and their contributions to complex "frontal lobe" tasks: A latent variable analysis. Cognitive Psychology. 2000;**41**(1):49-100

[34] Miyake A, Friedman NP. The nature and organization of individual differences in executive functions: Four general conclusions. Current Directions in Psychological Science. 2012;**21**(1):8-14

[35] Botvinick M, Braver T. Motivation and cognitive control: From behavior to neural mechanism. Annual Review of Psychology. 2015;**66**:83-113

[36] Ridderinkhof KR. Neurocognitive mechanisms of perception-action coordination: A review and theoretical integration. Neuroscience and Biobehavioral Reviews. 2014; **46**(Pt 1):3-29

[37] Verbruggen F. Executive control of actions across time and space. Current Directions in Psychological Science. 2016;**25**(6):399-404

[38] Verbruggen F, Logan GD. Proactive adjustments of response strategies in the stop-signal paradigm. Journal of Experimental Psychology. Human Perception and Performance. 2009;**35**(3):835-854

[39] Friedman NP, Miyake A. The relations among inhibition and interference control functions: A latent-variable analysis. Journal of Experimental Psychology. General. 2004;**133**(1):101-135

[40] Pettigrew C, Martin RC. Cognitive declines in healthy aging: Evidence from multiple aspects of interference resolution. Psychology and Aging. 2014;**29**(2):187-204

[41] Rey-Mermet A, Gade M, Oberauer K. Should we stop thinking about inhibition? Searching for individual and age differences in inhibition ability. Journal of Experimental Psychology. Learning, Memory, and Cognition. 2018;**44**(4):501-526

[42] Stahl C, Voss A, Schmitz F, Nuszbaum M, Tüscher O, Lieb K, et al. Behavioral components of impulsivity. Journal of Experimental Psychology. General. 2014;**143**(2):850-886

[43] Aron AR. From reactive to proactive and selective control: Developing a richer model for stopping inappropriate responses. Biological Psychiatry. 2011;**69**(12):e55-e68

[44] Braver TS. The variable nature of cognitive control: A dual mechanisms framework. Trends in Cognitive Sciences. 2012;**16**(2):106-113

[45] Zandbelt BB, Bloemendaal M, Neggers SFW, Kahn RS, Vink M. Expectations and violations: Delineating the neural network of proactive inhibitory control. Human Brain Mapping. 2013;**34**(9):2015-2024

[46] Schall JD, Godlove DC. Current advances and pressing problems in studies of stopping. Current Opinion in Neurobiology. 2012;**22**(6):1012-1021

[47] Fillmore MT, Weafer J. Behavioral inhibition and addiction. In: MacKillop J, de Wit H, editors. The Wiley-Blackwell Handbook of Addiction Psychopharmacology. Chichester, West Sussex; Malden, MA: Wiley-Blackwell; 2013. pp. 135-164

[48] Verdejo-Garcia A, Chong TT-J, Stout JC, Yücel M, London ED. Stages of dysfunctional decision-making in

addiction. Pharmacology, Biochemistry, and Behavior. 2018;**164**:99-105

[49] Billieux J, Gay P, Rochat L, Khazaal Y, Zullino D, Van der Linden M. Lack of inhibitory control predicts cigarette smoking dependence: Evidence from a non-deprived sample of light to moderate smokers. Drug and Alcohol Dependence. 2010;**112**(1-2):164-167

[50] Powell J, Dawkins L, West R, Powell J, Pickering A. Relapse to smoking during unaided cessation: Clinical, cognitive and motivational predictors. Psychopharmacology. 2010;**212**(4):537-549

[51] Noël X, Van der Linden M, Schmidt N, Sferrazza R, Hanak C, Le Bon O, et al. Supervisory attentional system in nonamnesic alcoholic men. Archives of General Psychiatry. 2001;**58**(12):1152-1158

[52] Noël X, Brevers D, Hanak C, Kornreich C, Verbanck P, Verbruggen F. On the automaticity of response inhibition in individuals with alcoholism. Journal of Behavior Therapy and Experimental Psychiatry. 2016;**51**:84-91

[53] Adams S, Mokrysz C, Attwood AS, Munafò MR. Resisting the urge to smoke: Inhibitory control training in cigarette smokers. Royal Society Open Science. 2017;**4**(8):170045

[54] Galimberti E, Martoni RM, Cavallini MC, Erzegovesi S, Bellodi L. Motor inhibition and cognitive flexibility in eating disorder subtypes. Progress in Neuro-Psychopharmacology & Biological Psychiatry. 2012;**36**(2):307-312

[55] Brevers D, Noël X. Pathological gambling and the loss of willpower: A neurocognitive perspective. Socioaffective Neuroscience & Psychology. 2013;**3**:21592

[56] Sharif-Razi M, Hodgins DC, Goghari VM. Reactive and proactive control mechanisms of response inhibition in gambling disorder. Psychiatry Research. 2019;**272**:114-121

[57] Czapla M, Simon JJ, Richter B, Kluge M, Friederich H-C, Herpertz S, et al. The impact of cognitive impairment and impulsivity on relapse of alcohol-dependent patients: Implications for psychotherapeutic treatment. Addiction Biology. 2016;**21**(4):873-884

[58] Goudriaan AE, Oosterlaan J, De Beurs E, Van Den Brink W. The role of self-reported impulsivity and reward sensitivity versus neurocognitive measures of disinhibition and decision-making in the prediction of relapse in pathological gamblers. Psychological Medicine. 2008;**38**(1):41-50

[59] Charles-Walsh K, Furlong L, Munro DG, Hester R. Inhibitory control dysfunction in nicotine dependence and the influence of short-term abstinence. Drug and Alcohol Dependence. 2014;**143**:81-86

[60] Smith JL, Mattick RP, Jamadar SD, Iredale JM. Deficits in behavioural inhibition in substance abuse and addiction: A meta-analysis. Drug and Alcohol Dependence. 2014;**145C**:1-33

[61] Otten R, Mun CJ, Shaw DS, Wilson MN, Dishion TJ. A developmental cascade model for early adolescent-onset substance use: The role of early childhood stress. Addiction. 2019;**114**(2):326-334

[62] Noël X, Bechara A, Dan B, Hanak C, Verbanck P. Response inhibition deficit is involved in poor decision making under risk in nonamnesic individuals with alcoholism. Neuropsychology. 2007;**21**(6):778-786

[63] Bechara A, Damasio H, Tranel D, Damasio AR. Deciding advantageously before knowing the advantageous strategy. Science. 1997;**275**(5304): 1293-1295

[64] Bechara A. Risky business: Emotion, decision-making, and addiction. Journal of Gambling Studies. 2003;**19**(1):23-51

[65] Bechara A. The role of emotion in decision-making: Evidence from neurological patients with orbitofrontal damage. Brain and Cognition. 2004;**55**(1):30-40

[66] Verbruggen F, Adams R, Chambers CD. Proactive motor control reduces monetary risk taking in gambling. Psychological Science. 2012;**23**(7):805-815

[67] Verbruggen F, Adams RC, van't Wout F, Stevens T, McLaren IPL, Chambers CD. Are the effects of response inhibition on gambling long-lasting? PLoS One. 2013;**8**(7):e70155

[68] Stevens T, Brevers D, Chambers CD, Lavric A, McLaren IPL, Mertens M, et al. How does response inhibition influence decision making when gambling? Journal of Experimental Psychology. Applied. 2015;**21**(1):15-36

[69] Stacy AW, Wiers RW. Implicit cognition and addiction: A tool for explaining paradoxical behavior. Annual Review of Clinical Psychology. 2010;**6**:551-575

[70] Houben K, Wiers RW. Response inhibition moderates the relationship between implicit associations and drinking behavior. Alcoholism, Clinical and Experimental Research. 2009;**33**(4):626-633

[71] Thush C, Wiers RW, Ames SL, Grenard JL, Sussman S, Stacy AW. Interactions between implicit and explicit cognition and working memory capacity in the prediction of alcohol use in at-risk adolescents. Drug and Alcohol Dependence. 2008;**94**(1-3):116-124

[72] Figner B, Knoch D, Johnson EJ, Krosch AR, Lisanby SH, Fehr E, et al. Lateral prefrontal cortex and self-control in intertemporal choice. Nature Neuroscience. 2010;**13**(5):538-539

[73] Kirby KN, Petry NM, Bickel WK. Heroin addicts have higher discount rates for delayed rewards than non-drug-using controls. Journal of Experimental Psychology. General. 1999;**128**(1):78-87

[74] Amlung M, Vedelago L, Acker J, Balodis I, MacKillop J. Steep delay discounting and addictive behavior: A meta-analysis of continuous associations. Addiction. 2017;**112**(1):51-62

[75] Bickel WK, Koffarnus MN, Moody L, Wilson AG. The behavioral- and neuro-economic process of temporal discounting: A candidate behavioral marker of addiction. Neuropharmacology. 2014; **76**(Pt B):518-527

[76] Bjork JM, Momenan R, Hommer DW. Delay discounting correlates with proportional lateral frontal cortex volumes. Biological Psychiatry. 2009;**65**(8):710-713

[77] Jauregi A, Kessler K, Hassel S. Linking cognitive measures of response inhibition and reward sensitivity to trait impulsivity. Frontiers in Psychology. 2018;**9**:2306

[78] Solanto MV, Abikoff H, Sonuga-Barke E, Schachar R, Logan GD, Wigal T, et al. The ecological validity of delay aversion and response inhibition as measures of impulsivity in AD/HD: A supplement to the NIMH multimodal treatment study of AD/HD. Journal of Abnormal Child Psychology. 2001;**29**(3):215-228

[79] Verdejo-Garcia A. Cognitive training for substance use disorders: Neuroscientific mechanisms. Neuroscience and Biobehavioral Reviews. 2016;**68**:270-281

[80] Enge S, Behnke A, Fleischhauer M, Küttler L, Kliegel M, Strobel A. No evidence for true training and transfer effects after inhibitory control training in young healthy adults. Journal of Experimental Psychology. Learning, Memory, and Cognition. 2014;**40**(4):987-1001

[81] Jones A, Guerrieri R, Fernie G, Cole J, Goudie A, Field M. The effects of priming restrained versus disinhibited behaviour on alcohol-seeking in social drinkers. Drug and Alcohol Dependence. 2011;**113**(1):55-61

[82] Redick TS, Shipstead Z, Harrison TL, Hicks KL, Fried DE, Hambrick DZ, et al. No evidence of intelligence improvement after working memory training: A randomized, placebo-controlled study. Journal of Experimental Psychology. General. 2013;**142**(2):359-379

[83] Klingberg T. Training and plasticity of working memory. Trends in Cognitive Sciences. 2010;**14**(7):317-324

[84] Houben K, Wiers RW, Jansen A. Getting a grip on drinking behavior: Training working memory to reduce alcohol abuse. Psychological Science. 2011;**22**(7):968-975

[85] Wanmaker S, Leijdesdorff SMJ, Geraerts E, van de Wetering BJM, Renkema PJ, Franken IHA. The efficacy of a working memory training in substance use patients: A randomized double-blind placebo-controlled clinical trial. Journal of Clinical and Experimental Neuropsychology. 2018;**40**(5):473-486

[86] Alcorn JL, Pike E, Stoops WS, Lile JA, Rush CR. A pilot investigation of acute inhibitory control training in cocaine users. Drug and Alcohol Dependence. 2017;**174**:145-149

[87] Houben K, Havermans RC, Nederkoorn C, Jansen A. Beer à no-go: Learning to stop responding to alcohol cues reduces alcohol intake via reduced affective associations rather than increased response inhibition. Addiction. 2012;**107**(7):1280-1287

[88] Houben K, Jansen A. Training inhibitory control. A recipe for resisting sweet temptations. Appetite. 2011;**56**(2):345-349

[89] Jones A, Di Lemma LCG, Robinson E, Christiansen P, Nolan S, Tudur-Smith C, et al. Inhibitory control training for appetitive behaviour change: A meta-analytic investigation of mechanisms of action and moderators of effectiveness. Appetite. 2016;**97**:16-28

[90] Jones A, Field M. The effects of cue-specific inhibition training on alcohol consumption in heavy social drinkers. Experimental and Clinical Psychopharmacology. 2013;**21**(1):8-16

[91] Allom V, Mullan B, Hagger M. Does inhibitory control training improve health behaviour? A meta-analysis. Health Psychology Review. 2016;**10**(2):168-186

[92] Turton R, Bruidegom K, Cardi V, Hirsch CR, Treasure J. Novel methods to help develop healthier eating habits for eating and weight disorders: A systematic review and meta-analysis. Neuroscience and Biobehavioral Reviews. 2016;**61**:132-155

[93] Eagle DM, Bari A, Robbins TW. The neuropsychopharmacology of action inhibition: Cross-species translation of the stop-signal and go/no-go tasks. Psychopharmacology. 2008;**199**(3):439-456

[94] Verbruggen F, Logan GD. Automatic and controlled response inhibition: Associative learning in the go/no-go and stop-signal paradigms. Journal of Experimental Psychology. General. 2008;**137**(4):649-672

[95] Adams RC, Lawrence NS, Verbruggen F, Chambers CD. Training response inhibition to reduce food consumption: Mechanisms, stimulus specificity and appropriate training protocols. Appetite. 2017;**109**:11-23

[96] Lawrence NS, Verbruggen F, Morrison S, Adams RC, Chambers CD. Stopping to food can reduce intake. Effects of stimulus-specificity and individual differences in dietary restraint. Appetite. 2015;**85**:91-103

[97] Lapenta OM, Sierve KD, de Macedo EC, Fregni F, Boggio PS. Transcranial direct current stimulation modulates ERP-indexed inhibitory control and reduces food consumption. Appetite. 2014;**83**:42-48

[98] Veling H, Aarts H, Papies EK. Using stop signals to inhibit chronic dieters' responses toward palatable foods. Behaviour Research and Therapy. 2011;**49**(11):771-780

[99] Hare TA, Camerer CF, Rangel A. Self-control in decision-making involves modulation of the vmPFC valuation system. Science. New York, N.Y. 2009;**324**(5927):646-648

[100] Veling H, Aarts H, Stroebe W. Stop signals decrease choices for palatable foods through decreased food evaluation. Frontiers in Psychology. 2013;**4**:875

[101] Wessel JR, O'Doherty JP, Berkebile MM, Linderman D, Aron AR. Stimulus devaluation induced by stopping action. Journal of Experimental Psychology. General. 2014;**143**(6):2316-2329

[102] Friese M, Hofmann W, Wänke M. When impulses take over: Moderated predictive validity of explicit and implicit attitude measures in predicting food choice and consumption behaviour. The British Journal of Social Psychology. 2008;**47**(Pt 3):397-419

[103] Ferrey AE, Frischen A, Fenske MJ. Hot or not: Response inhibition reduces the hedonic value and motivational incentive of sexual stimuli. Frontiers in Psychology. 2012;**3**:575

[104] Lawrence NS, O'Sullivan J, Parslow D, Javaid M, Adams RC, Chambers CD, et al. Training response inhibition to food is associated with weight loss and reduced energy intake. Appetite. 2015;**95**:17-28

[105] Veling H, Holland RW, van Knippenberg A. When approach motivation and behavioral inhibition collide: Behavior regulation through stimulus devaluation. Journal of Experimental Social Psychology. 2008;**44**(4):1013-1019

[106] Eberl C, Wiers RW, Pawelczack S, Rinck M, Becker ES, Lindenmeyer J. Approach bias modification in alcohol dependence: Do clinical effects replicate and for whom does it work best? Developmental Cognitive Neuroscience. 2013;**4**:38-51

[107] Wiers RW, Eberl C, Rinck M, Becker ES, Lindenmeyer J. Retraining automatic action tendencies changes alcoholic patients' approach bias for alcohol and improves treatment outcome. Psychological Science. 2011;**22**(4):490-497

[108] Cristea IA, Kok RN, Cuijpers P. The effectiveness of cognitive bias modification interventions for substance addictions: A meta-analysis. PLoS One. 2016;**11**(9):e0162226

[109] Wiers RW, Boffo M, Field M. What's in a trial? On the importance of distinguishing between experimental lab studies and randomized controlled trials: The case of cognitive bias modification and alcohol use disorders.

Journal of Studies on Alcohol and Drugs. 2018;**79**(3):333-343

[110] Boffo M, Pronk T, Wiers RW, Mannarini S. Combining cognitive bias modification training with motivational support in alcohol dependent outpatients: Study protocol for a randomised controlled trial. Trials. 2015;**16**:63

[111] Houben K, Havermans RC, Wiers RW. Learning to dislike alcohol: Conditioning negative implicit attitudes toward alcohol and its effect on drinking behavior. Psychopharmacology. 2010;**211**(1):79-86

[112] Freeman SM, Razhas I, Aron AR. Top-down response suppression mitigates action tendencies triggered by a motivating stimulus. Current Biology: CB. 2014;**24**(2):212-216

[113] Veling H, Aarts H, Stroebe W. Using stop signals to reduce impulsive choices for palatable unhealthy foods. British Journal of Health Psychology. 2013;**18**(2):354-368

[114] Rolland B, D'Hondt F, Montègue S, Brion M, Peyron E, D'Aviau de Ternay J, et al. A patient-tailored evidence-based approach for developing early neuropsychological training programs in addiction settings. Neuropsychology Review. 2019;**29**(1):103-115

[115] Kuhn J, Lenartz D, Huff W, Lee S, Koulousakis A, Klosterkoetter J, et al. Remission of alcohol dependency following deep brain stimulation of the nucleus accumbens: Valuable therapeutic implications? Journal of Neurology, Neurosurgery, and Psychiatry. 2007;**78**(10):1152-1153

[116] Levy D, Shabat-Simon M, Shalev U, Barnea-Ygael N, Cooper A, Zangen A. Repeated electrical stimulation of reward-related brain regions affects cocaine but not "natural" reinforcement. The Journal of Neuroscience. 2007;**27**(51): 14179-14189

[117] Voges J, Waerzeggers Y, Maarouf M, Lehrke R, Koulousakis A, Lenartz D, et al. Deep-brain stimulation: Long-term analysis of complications caused by hardware and surgery—Experiences from a single centre. Journal of Neurology, Neurosurgery, and Psychiatry. 2006;**77**(7):868-872

[118] Wang TR, Moosa S, Dallapiazza RF, Elias WJ, Lynch WJ. Deep brain stimulation for the treatment of drug addiction. Neurosurgical Focus. 2018;**45**(2):E11

[119] Benabid AL, Pollak P, Louveau A, Henry S, de Rougemont J. Combined (thalamotomy and stimulation) stereotactic surgery of the VIM thalamic nucleus for bilateral Parkinson disease. Applied Neurophysiology. 1987;**50**(1-6):344-346

[120] Nuttin B, Cosyns P, Demeulemeester H, Gybels J, Meyerson B. Electrical stimulation in anterior limbs of internal capsules in patients with obsessive-compulsive disorder. The Lancet. 1999;**354**(9189):1526

[121] Mayberg HS, Lozano AM, Voon V, McNeely HE, Seminowicz D, Hamani C, et al. Deep brain stimulation for treatment-resistant depression. Neuron. 2005;**45**(5):651-660

[122] Kuhn J, Bauer R, Pohl S, Lenartz D, Huff W, Kim EH, et al. Observations on unaided smoking cessation after deep brain stimulation of the nucleus accumbens. European Addiction Research. 2009;**15**(4):196-201

[123] Ardouin C, Voon V, Worbe Y, Abouazar N, Czernecki V, Hosseini H, et al. Pathological gambling in Parkinson's disease improves on chronic subthalamic nucleus stimulation. Movement Disorders. 2006;**21**(11):1941-1946

[124] Luigjes J, Segrave R, de Joode N, Figee M, Denys D. Efficacy of invasive and non-invasive brain modulation interventions for addiction. Neuropsychology Review. 2018;**29**:116-138

[125] Sesia T, Bulthuis V, Tan S, Lim LW, Vlamings R, Blokland A, et al. Deep brain stimulation of the nucleus accumbens shell increases impulsive behavior and tissue levels of dopamine and serotonin. Experimental Neurology. 2010;**225**(2):302-309

[126] Sesia T, Temel Y, Lim LW, Blokland A, Steinbusch HWM, Visser-Vandewalle V. Deep brain stimulation of the nucleus accumbens core and shell: Opposite effects on impulsive action. Experimental Neurology. 2008;**214**(1):135-139

[127] Crews FT, Boettiger CA. Impulsivity, frontal lobes and risk for addiction. Pharmacology, Biochemistry, and Behavior. 2009;**93**(3):237-247

[128] Luigjes J, van den Brink W, Schuurman PR, Kuhn J, Denys D. Is deep brain stimulation a treatment option for addiction? Addiction. 2015;**110**(4):547-548

[129] Kekic M, Boysen E, Campbell IC, Schmidt U. A systematic review of the clinical efficacy of transcranial direct current stimulation (tDCS) in psychiatric disorders. Journal of Psychiatric Research. 2016;**74**:70-86

[130] Tortella G. Transcranial direct current stimulation in psychiatric disorders. World Journal of Psychiatry. 2015;**5**(1):88

[131] Jansen JM, Daams JG, Koeter MWJ, Veltman DJ, van den Brink W, Goudriaan AE. Effects of non-invasive neurostimulation on craving: A meta-analysis. Neuroscience & Biobehavioral Reviews. 2013;**37**(10):2472-2480

[132] Chen R, Classen J, Gerloff C, Celnik P, Wassermann EM, Hallett M, et al. Depression of motor cortex excitability by low-frequency transcranial magnetic stimulation. Neurology. 1997;**48**(5):1398-1403

[133] Siebner HR, Peller M, Willoch F, Minoshima S, Boecker H, Auer C, et al. Lasting cortical activation after repetitive TMS of the motor cortex: A glucose metabolic study. Neurology. 2000;**54**(4):956-963

[134] Maeda F, Keenan JP, Tormos JM, Topka H, Pascual-Leone A. Interindividual variability of the modulatory effects of repetitive transcranial magnetic stimulation on cortical excitability. Experimental Brain Research. 2000;**133**(4):425-430

[135] Deng Z-D, Lisanby SH, Peterchev AV. Electric field depth-focality tradeoff in transcranial magnetic stimulation: Simulation comparison of 50 coil designs. Brain Stimulation. 2013;**6**(1):1-13

[136] Amiaz R, Levy D, Vainiger D, Grunhaus L, Zangen A. Repeated high-frequency transcranial magnetic stimulation over the dorsolateral prefrontal cortex reduces cigarette craving and consumption. Addiction. 2009;**104**(4):653-660

[137] Trojak B, Meille V, Achab S, Lalanne L, Poquet H, Ponavoy E, et al. Transcranial magnetic stimulation combined with nicotine replacement therapy for smoking cessation: A randomized controlled trial. Brain Stimulation. 2015;**8**(6):1168-1174

[138] Ceccanti M, Inghilleri M, Attilia ML, Raccah R, Fiore M, Zangen A, et al. Deep TMS on alcoholics: Effects on cortisolemia and dopamine pathway modulation. A pilot study. Canadian Journal of Physiology and Pharmacology. 2015;**93**(4):283-290

[139] Bolloni C, Panella R, Pedetti M, Frascella AG, Gambelunghe C, Piccoli T, et al. Bilateral transcranial magnetic stimulation of the prefrontal cortex reduces cocaine intake: A pilot study. Frontiers in Psychiatry. 2016;**7**:133

[140] Höppner J, Broese T, Wendler L, Berger C, Thome J. Repetitive transcranial magnetic stimulation (rTMS) for treatment of alcohol dependence. The World Journal of Biological Psychiatry. 2011; **12**(Suppl 1):57-62

[141] Herremans SC, Vanderhasselt M-A, De Raedt R, Baeken C. Reduced intra-individual reaction time variability during a Go-NoGo task in detoxified alcohol-dependent patients after one right-sided dorsolateral prefrontal HF-rTMS session. Alcohol and Alcoholism (Oxford, Oxfordshire). 2013;**48**(5):552-557

[142] Steele JD, Lawrie SM. Segregation of cognitive and emotional function in the prefrontal cortex: A stereotactic meta-analysis. NeuroImage. 2004;**21**(3):868-875

[143] Naqvi NH, Rudrauf D, Damasio H, Bechara A. Damage to the insula disrupts addiction to cigarette smoking. Science. 2007;**315**(5811):531-534

[144] Volkow ND, Baler RD. NOW vs LATER brain circuits: Implications for obesity and addiction. Trends in Neurosciences. 2015;**38**(6):345-352

[145] Cho SS, Koshimori Y, Aminian K, Obeso I, Rusjan P, Lang AE, et al. Investing in the future: Stimulation of the medial prefrontal cortex reduces discounting of delayed rewards. Neuropsychopharmacology. 2015;**40**(3):546-553

[146] Zack M, Cho SS, Parlee J, Jacobs M, Li C, Boileau I, et al. Effects of high frequency repeated transcranial magnetic stimulation and continuous theta burst stimulation on gambling reinforcement, delay discounting, and stroop interference in men with pathological gambling. Brain Stimulation. 2016;**9**(6):867-875

[147] Huang Y-Z, Edwards MJ, Rounis E, Bhatia KP, Rothwell JC. Theta burst stimulation of the human motor cortex. Neuron. 2005;**45**(2):201-206

[148] Lowe CJ, Manocchio F, Safati AB, Hall PA. The effects of theta burst stimulation (TBS) targeting the prefrontal cortex on executive functioning: A systematic review and meta-analysis. Neuropsychologia. 2018;**111**:344-359

[149] Nitsche MA, Paulus W. Excitability changes induced in the human motor cortex by weak transcranial direct current stimulation. The Journal of Physiology. 2000;**527**(Pt 3):633-639

[150] Nitsche MA, Paulus W. Sustained excitability elevations induced by transcranial DC motor cortex stimulation in humans. Neurology. 2001;**57**(10):1899-1901

[151] Woods AJ, Antal A, Bikson M, Boggio PS, Brunoni AR, Celnik P, et al. A technical guide to tDCS, and related non-invasive brain stimulation tools. Clinical Neurophysiology. 2016;**127**(2):1031-1048

[152] Boggio PS, Nunes A, Rigonatti SP, Nitsche MA, Pascual-Leone A, Fregni F. Repeated sessions of noninvasive brain DC stimulation is associated with motor function improvement in stroke patients. Restorative Neurology and Neuroscience. 2007;**25**(2):123-129

[153] Strube W, Bunse T, Nitsche MA, Nikolaeva A, Palm U, Padberg F, et al. Bidirectional variability in motor cortex excitability modulation following 1 mA

transcranial direct current stimulation in healthy participants. Physiological Reports. 2016;**4**(15):e12884

[154] Kang N, Kim RK, Kim HJ. Effects of transcranial direct current stimulation on symptoms of nicotine dependence: A systematic review and meta-analysis. Addictive Behaviors. 2019;**96**:133-139

[155] Sauvaget A, Trojak B, Bulteau S, Jiménez-Murcia S, Fernández-Aranda F, Wolz I, et al. Transcranial direct current stimulation (tDCS) in behavioral and food addiction: A systematic review of efficacy, technical, and methodological issues. Frontiers in Neuroscience. 2015;**9**:349

[156] Spagnolo PA, Goldman D. Neuromodulation interventions for addictive disorders: Challenges, promise, and roadmap for future research. Brain. 2017;**140**(5):1183-1203

[157] Russo R, Twyman P, Cooper NR, Fitzgerald PB, Wallace D. When you can, scale up: Large-scale study shows no effect of tDCS in an ambiguous risk-taking task. Neuropsychologia. 2017;**104**:133-143

[158] Skinner MD, Aubin H-J. Craving's place in addiction theory: Contributions of the major models. Neuroscience and Biobehavioral Reviews. 2010;**34**(4):606-623

[159] Klauss J, Penido Pinheiro LC, Silva Merlo BL, Santos GAC, Fregni F, Nitsche MA, et al. A randomized controlled trial of targeted prefrontal cortex modulation with tDCS in patients with alcohol dependence. The International Journal of Neuropsychopharmacology. 2014;**17**(11):1793-1803

[160] Falcone M, Bernardo L, Wileyto EP, Allenby C, Burke AM, Hamilton R, et al. Lack of effect of transcranial direct current stimulation (tDCS) on short-term smoking cessation: Results of a randomized, sham-controlled clinical trial. Drug and Alcohol Dependence. 2019;**194**:244-251

[161] Mondino M, Luck D, Grot S, Januel D, Suaud-Chagny M-F, Poulet E, et al. Effects of repeated transcranial direct current stimulation on smoking, craving and brain reactivity to smoking cues. Scientific Reports. 2018;**8**(1):8724

[162] Fregni F, Orsati F, Pedrosa W, Fecteau S, Tome FAM, Nitsche MA, et al. Transcranial direct current stimulation of the prefrontal cortex modulates the desire for specific foods. Appetite. 2008;**51**(1):34-41

[163] Goldman RL, Borckardt JJ, Frohman HA, O'Neil PM, Madan A, Campbell LK, et al. Prefrontal cortex transcranial direct current stimulation (tDCS) temporarily reduces food cravings and increases the self-reported ability to resist food in adults with frequent food craving. Appetite. 2011;**56**(3):741-746

[164] Kekic M, McClelland J, Campbell I, Nestler S, Rubia K, David AS, et al. The effects of prefrontal cortex transcranial direct current stimulation (tDCS) on food craving and temporal discounting in women with frequent food cravings. Appetite. 2014;**78**:55-62

[165] Montenegro RA, Okano AH, Cunha FA, Gurgel JL, Fontes EB, Farinatti PTV. Prefrontal cortex transcranial direct current stimulation associated with aerobic exercise change aspects of appetite sensation in overweight adults. Appetite. 2012;**58**(1):333-338

[166] Keeser D, Meindl T, Bor J, Palm U, Pogarell O, Mulert C, et al. Prefrontal transcranial direct current stimulation changes connectivity

of resting-state networks during fMRI. The Journal of Neuroscience. 2011;**31**(43):15284-15293

[167] Meinzer M, Lindenberg R, Antonenko D, Flaisch T, Flöel A. Anodal transcranial direct current stimulation temporarily reverses age-associated cognitive decline and functional brain activity changes. The Journal of Neuroscience: The Official Journal of the Society for Neuroscience. 2013;**33**(30):12470-12478

[168] Nelson JT, McKinley RA, Golob EJ, Warm JS, Parasuraman R. Enhancing vigilance in operators with prefrontal cortex transcranial direct current stimulation (tDCS). NeuroImage. 2014;**85**(Pt 3):909-917

[169] Brunoni AR, Vanderhasselt M-A. Working memory improvement with non-invasive brain stimulation of the dorsolateral prefrontal cortex: A systematic review and meta-analysis. Brain and Cognition. 2014;**86**:1-9

[170] Cunillera T, Brignani D, Cucurell D, Fuentemilla L, Miniussi C. The right inferior frontal cortex in response inhibition: A tDCS-ERP co-registration study. NeuroImage. 2016;**140**:66-75

[171] Yu J, Tseng P, Hung DL, Wu S-W, Juan C-H. Brain stimulation improves cognitive control by modulating medial-frontal activity and preSMA-vmPFC functional connectivity. Human Brain Mapping. 2015;**36**(10):4004-4015

[172] Campanella S, Schroder E, Monnart A, Vanderhasselt M-A, Duprat R, Rabijns M, et al. Transcranial direct current stimulation over the right frontal inferior cortex decreases neural activity needed to achieve inhibition: A double-blind ERP study in a male population. Clinical EEG and Neuroscience. 2017;**48**(3):176-188

[173] Petit G, Cimochowska A, Kornreich C, Hanak C, Verbanck P, Campanella S. Neurophysiological correlates of response inhibition predict relapse in detoxified alcoholic patients: Some preliminary evidence from event-related potentials. Neuropsychiatric Disease and Treatment. 2014;**10**:1025-1037

[174] Osimo SA, Korb S, Aiello M. Obesity, subliminal perception and inhibition: Neuromodulation of the prefrontal cortex. Behaviour Research and Therapy. 2019;**119**:103408

[175] Dickerson KC. Upregulating brain activity using non-drug reward imagery and real-time fMRI neurofeedback—A new treatment approach for addiction? eBioMedicine. 2018;**38**:21-22

[176] Orndorff-Plunkett F, Singh F, Aragón OR, Pineda JA. Assessing the effectiveness of neurofeedback training in the context of clinical and social neuroscience. Brain Sciences. 2017;**7**(8):95

[177] Thibault RT, Lifshitz M, Raz A. The self-regulating brain and neurofeedback: Experimental science and clinical promise. Cortex. 2016;**74**:247-261

[178] Cox WM, Subramanian L, Linden DEJ, Lührs M, McNamara R, Playle R, et al. Neurofeedback training for alcohol dependence versus treatment as usual: Study protocol for a randomized controlled trial. Trials. 2016;**17**(1):480

[179] deCharms RC. Applications of real-time fMRI. Nature Reviews Neuroscience. 2008;**9**(9):720-729

[180] Hanlon CA, Hartwell KJ, Canterberry M, Li X, Owens M, LeMatty T, et al. Reduction of cue-induced craving through realtime neurofeedback in nicotine users: The role of region of interest selection and multiple visits. Psychiatry Research: Neuroimaging. 2013;**213**(1):79-81

[181] Sitaram R, Ros T, Stoeckel L, Haller S, Scharnowski F, Lewis-Peacock J, et al. Closed-loop brain training: The science of neurofeedback. Nature Reviews Neuroscience. 2017;**18**(2):86-100

[182] Scott WC, Kaiser D, Othmer S, Sideroff SI. Effects of an EEG biofeedback protocol on a mixed substance abusing population. The American Journal of Drug and Alcohol Abuse. 2005;**31**(3):455-469

[183] Keith JR, Rapgay L, Theodore D, Schwartz JM, Ross JL. An assessment of an automated EEG biofeedback system for attention deficits in a substance use disorders residential treatment setting. Psychology of Addictive Behaviors. 2015;**29**(1):17-25

[184] Kober SE, Witte M, Stangl M, Väljamäe A, Neuper C, Wood G. Shutting down sensorimotor interference unblocks the networks for stimulus processing: An SMR neurofeedback training study. Clinical Neurophysiology. 2015;**126**(1):82-95

[185] Canterberry M, Hanlon CA, Hartwell KJ, Li X, Owens M, LeMatty T, et al. Sustained reduction of nicotine craving with real-time neurofeedback: Exploring the role of severity of dependence. Nicotine & Tobacco Research: Official Journal of the Society for Research on Nicotine and Tobacco. 2013;**15**(12):2120-2124

[186] Karch S, Paolini M, Gschwendtner S, Jeanty H, Reckenfelderbäumer A, Yaseen O, et al. Real-time fMRI neurofeedback in patients with tobacco use disorder during smoking cessation: Functional differences and implications of the first training session in regard to future abstinence or relapse. Frontiers in Human Neuroscience. 2019;**13**:65

[187] Lapenta OM, Marques LM, Rego GG, Comfort WE, Boggio PS. tDCS in addiction and impulse control disorders. The Journal of ECT. 2018;**34**(3):182-192

[188] Sathappan AV, Luber BM, Lisanby SH. The dynamic duo: Combining noninvasive brain stimulation with cognitive interventions. Progress in Neuro-Psychopharmacology & Biological Psychiatry. 2019;**89**:347-360

[189] Rabey JM, Dobronevsky E, Aichenbaum S, Gonen O, Marton RG, Khaigrekht M. Repetitive transcranial magnetic stimulation combined with cognitive training is a safe and effective modality for the treatment of Alzheimer's disease: A randomized, double-blind study. Journal of Neural Transmission. 2013;**120**(5):813-819

[190] Segrave RA, Arnold S, Hoy K, Fitzgerald PB. Concurrent cognitive control training augments the antidepressant efficacy of tDCS: A pilot study. Brain Stimulation. 2014;**7**(2):325-331

[191] den Uyl TE, Gladwin TE, Wiers RW. Electrophysiological and behavioral effects of combined transcranial direct current stimulation and alcohol approach bias retraining in hazardous drinkers. Alcoholism, Clinical and Experimental Research. 2016;**40**(10):2124-2133

[192] den Uyl TE, Gladwin TE, Rinck M, Lindenmeyer J, Wiers RW. A clinical trial with combined transcranial direct current stimulation and alcohol approach bias retraining. Addiction Biology. 2017;**22**(6):1632-1640

[193] den Uyl TE, Gladwin TE, Lindenmeyer J, Wiers RW. A clinical trial with combined transcranial direct current stimulation and attentional bias modification in alcohol-dependent patients. Alcoholism, Clinical and Experimental Research. 2018;**42**(10):1961-1969

[194] Sedgmond J, Lawrence NS, Verbruggen F, Morrison S, Chambers CD, Adams RC. Prefrontal brain stimulation during food-related inhibition training: Effects on food craving, food consumption and inhibitory control. Royal Society Open Science. 2019;**6**(1):181186

[195] Claus ED, Klimaj SD, Chavez R, Martinez AD, Clark VP. A randomized trial of combined tDCS over right inferior frontal cortex and cognitive bias modification: Null effects on drinking and alcohol approach bias. Alcoholism, Clinical and Experimental Research. 2019;**43**(7):1591-1599

[196] Heeren A, Billieux J, Philippot P, De Raedt R, Baeken C, de Timary P, et al. Impact of transcranial direct current stimulation on attentional bias for threat: A proof-of-concept study among individuals with social anxiety disorder. Social Cognitive and Affective Neuroscience. 2017;**12**(2):251-260

[197] Carmi L, Tendler A, Bystritsky A, Hollander E, Blumberger DM, Daskalakis J, et al. Efficacy and safety of deep transcranial magnetic stimulation for obsessive-compulsive disorder: A prospective multicenter randomized double-blind placebo-controlled trial. The American Journal of Psychiatry. 21 May 2019

[198] Carmi L, Alyagon U, Barnea-Ygael N, Zohar J, Dar R, Zangen A. Clinical and electrophysiological outcomes of deep TMS over the medial prefrontal and anterior cingulate cortices in OCD patients. Brain Stimulation. 2018;**11**(1):158-165

[199] Dinur-Klein L, Dannon P, Hadar A, Rosenberg O, Roth Y, Kotler M, et al. Smoking cessation induced by deep repetitive transcranial magnetic stimulation of the prefrontal and insular cortices: A prospective, randomized controlled trial. Biological Psychiatry. 2014;**76**(9):742-749

[200] Pavlov I. Conditioned Reflexes. USA: Oxford University Press; 1927

[201] Conklin CA, Tiffany ST. Applying extinction research and theory to cue-exposure addiction treatments. Addiction. 2002;**97**(2):155-167

[202] Dunsmoor JE, Niv Y, Daw N, Phelps EA. Rethinking extinction. Neuron. 2015;**88**(1):47-63

[203] Milton AL, Everitt BJ. The psychological and neurochemical mechanisms of drug memory reconsolidation: Implications for the treatment of addiction. The European Journal of Neuroscience. 2010;**31**(12):2308-2319

[204] Lee JLC, Nader K, Schiller D. An update on memory reconsolidation updating. Trends in Cognitive Sciences. 2017;**21**(7):531-545

[205] Nader K, Schafe GE, Le Doux JE. Fear memories require protein synthesis in the amygdala for reconsolidation after retrieval. Nature. 2000;**406**(6797):722-726

[206] Sandrini M, Cohen LG, Censor N. Modulating reconsolidation: A link to causal systems-level dynamics of human memories. Trends in Cognitive Sciences. 2015;**19**(8):475-482

[207] McGaugh JL. Time-dependent processes in memory storage. Science (New York, N.Y.). 1966;**153**(3742):1351-1358

[208] Soeter M, Kindt M. An abrupt transformation of phobic behavior after a post-retrieval amnesic agent. Biological Psychiatry. 2015;**78**(12):880-886

[209] Monfils M-H, Cowansage KK, Klann E, LeDoux JE. Extinction-reconsolidation boundaries: Key to persistent attenuation of fear memories. Science. 2009;**324**(5929):951-955

[210] Xue Y-X, Luo Y-X, Wu P, Shi H-S, Xue L-F, Chen C, et al. A memory retrieval-extinction procedure to prevent drug craving and relapse. Science (New York, N.Y.). 2012;**336**(6078):241-245

[211] Schiller D, Kanen JW, LeDoux JE, Monfils M-H, Phelps EA. Extinction during reconsolidation of threat memory diminishes prefrontal cortex involvement. Proceedings of the National Academy of Sciences of the United States of America. 2013;**110**(50):20040-20045

[212] Pedreira ME, Pérez-Cuesta LM, Maldonado H. Mismatch between what is expected and what actually occurs triggers memory reconsolidation or extinction. Learning & Memory (Cold Spring Harbor, N.Y.). 2004;**11**(5):579-585

[213] Sevenster D, Beckers T, Kindt M. Prediction error governs pharmacologically induced amnesia for learned fear. Science. 2013;**339**(6121):830-833

[214] Das RK, Lawn W, Kamboj SK. Rewriting the valuation and salience of alcohol-related stimuli via memory reconsolidation. Translational Psychiatry. 2015;**5**:e645

[215] Hon T, Das RK, Kamboj SK. The effects of cognitive reappraisal following retrieval-procedures designed to destabilize alcohol memories in high-risk drinkers. Psychopharmacology. 2016;**233**(5):851-861

[216] Kaag AM, Goudriaan AE, De Vries TJ, Pattij T, Wiers RW. A high working memory load prior to memory retrieval reduces craving in non-treatment seeking problem drinkers. Psychopharmacology. 2018;**235**(3):695-708

[217] Everitt BJ, Giuliano C, Belin D. Addictive behaviour in experimental animals: Prospects for translation. Philosophical Transactions of the Royal Society of London. Series B, Biological Sciences. 2018;**373**:1742

[218] Lane RD, Ryan L, Nadel L, Greenberg L. Memory reconsolidation, emotional arousal, and the process of change in psychotherapy: New insights from brain science. The Behavioral and Brain Sciences. 2015;**38**:e1

[219] Marián M, Szőllősi Á, Racsmány M. Anodal transcranial direct current stimulation of the right dorsolateral prefrontal cortex impairs long-term retention of reencountered memories. Cortex; A Journal Devoted to the Study of the Nervous System and Behavior. 2018;**108**:80-91

[220] Gladwin TE, Wiers CE, Wiers RW. Interventions aimed at automatic processes in addiction: Considering necessary conditions for efficacy. Current Opinion in Behavioral Sciences. 2017;**13**:19-24

[221] Connolly Gibbons MB, Crits-Christoph P, Barber JP, Stirman SW, Gallop R, Goldstein LA, et al. Unique and common mechanisms of change across cognitive and dynamic psychotherapies. Journal of Consulting and Clinical Psychology. 2009;**77**(5):801-813

[222] Connolly Gibbons MB, Crits-Christoph P, Barber JP, Schamberger M. Insight in psychotherapy: A review of empirical literature. In: Castonguay LG, Hill C, editors. Insight in Psychotherapy. 2007. pp. 143-165

[223] Gollwitzer P, Sheeran P. Implementation intentions and goal achievement: A meta-analysis of effects and processes. In: Zanna MP, editor. Advances in Experimental Social Psychology. Vol. 38. Academic Press; 2006. pp. 69-119

[224] Ekhtiari H, Tavakoli H, Addolorato G, Baeken C, Bonci A, Campanella S, et al. Transcranial electrical and magnetic stimulation (tES and TMS) for addiction medicine: A consensus paper on the present state of the science and the road ahead. Neuroscience and Biobehavioral Reviews. 2019;**104**:118-140

[225] Campanella S, Schroder E, Kajosch H, Noel X, Kornreich C. Why cognitive event-related potentials (ERPs) should have a role in the management of alcohol disorders. Neuroscience and Biobehavioral Reviews. San Diego, California. 21 Jun 2018

[226] Dunbar AB, Taylor JR. Reconsolidation and psychopathology: Moving towards reconsolidation-based treatments. Neurobiology of Learning and Memory. 2017;**142**(Pt A):162-171

[227] Monfils MH, Holmes EA. Memory boundaries: Opening a window inspired by reconsolidation to treat anxiety, trauma-related, and addiction disorders. The Lancet. Psychiatry. 2018;**5**(12):1032-1042

Chapter 4

Binge Drinking and Memory in Adolescents and Young Adults

Concepción Vinader-Caerols and Santiago Monleón

Abstract

The binge drinking (BD) pattern of alcohol consumption, characterized by intermittent consumption of large quantities of alcohol in short periods, is currently prevalent during adolescence and early youth. This period is characterized by critical changes to the structural and functional development of brain areas related with memory, as well as other executive functions. As a result, BD has been associated with undermined learning and memory ability in adolescents and youths of both sexes. One distinctive contribution of this chapter is to evaluate, together, the impact of an acute BD episode, the sample's history of consumption, and its effect on learning and memory performance and as potential gender differences. The main findings of the published research show that BD has differential effects on several types of memory and confirm that women are more vulnerable to these detrimental effects of alcohol than are men. These cognitive differences between men and women seem to be overridden as the blood alcohol concentration progressively increases. As BD pattern of consumption has been associated with inhibitory control deficits, future research also should investigate long-term implementation of inhibitory control training, emphasizing the importance of this training as part of the intervention strategies focused on this at-risk group.

Keywords: binge drinking, memory, adolescence, youth, gender

1. Introduction

Alcohol is one of the most widely consumed psychoactive substances in the world, especially among adolescents and young adults [1, 2]. Many of these develop a pattern of alcohol consumption known as binge drinking (BD). BD has been defined by The National Institute on Alcohol Abuse and Alcoholism (NIAAA) as a pattern of drinking that elevates a person's blood alcohol concentration (BAC) to 0.8 g/L or above [3]. This pattern involves the intake of large quantities of alcohol in a short period (about 2 h), followed by a period of abstinence, with a variability between 1 week and 1 month (see **Figure 1**). BD is the most common pattern of alcohol use among adolescents and young adults in Western countries. In Spain, the prevalence of BD pattern is similar in both sexes among 14–16 year-old adolescents and is more widespread among men than women in the age range of 17–18 years [4].

Individuals engaging in frequent BD have an increased risk to develop an alcohol use disorder (AUD) later in life. This risk has been suggested to be linked to

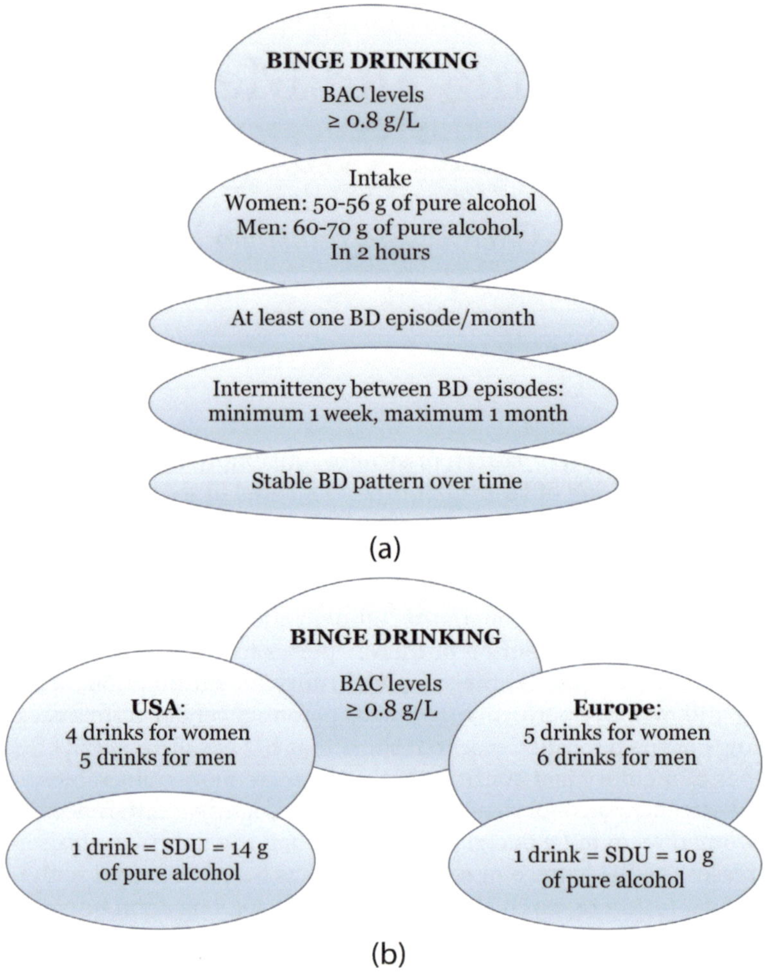

Figure 1.
(a) Binge drinking pattern criteria. Quantity: intake of 50–56 g of pure alcohol in women and 60–70 g in men, in 2 h. Frequency: at least one BD episode per month. Intermittency: abstinence between BD episodes over time (minimum 1 week, maximum 1 month). (b) Number of drinks (1 drink = SDU, standard drink unit) in the USA and Europe for binge drinking's BAC levels.

executive deficits (e.g., [5]). The BD pattern of consumption seems to be especially associated with increased impulsivity and inhibitory control deficits (e.g., [6–8]). At the same time, this seems to be due to an attenuated frontal activation (e.g., [8, 9]). Thus, a higher incidence of BD has been related to decreased activation of dorsolateral prefrontal cortex, dorsomedial prefrontal cortex, and anterior cingulate cortex, brain regions strongly implicated in executive functioning [9]. The neurotoxic effects of BD on these regions can be less evident throughout adolescence, but if this alcohol consumption pattern persists, the executive dysfunction could be exacerbated. While individuals with AUD typically exhibit inhibitory control dysfunction, evidence of impaired inhibitory control among binge drinkers, who are at increased risk of developing an AUD, is mixed. Despite the variability in the literature, some findings point to mechanisms that may confer vulnerability for transition from binge drinking to AUD [6]. Therefore, inhibitory control deficits must be considered as an important factor that contributes to alcohol abuse.

On the other hand, important physical, social, and cognitive skills are acquired during adolescence and early youth. This period is also characterized by critical changes to the structural and functional development of brain areas related with these skills [10]. For example, the superior associative cortex (e.g., prefrontal cortex) undergoes myelination, pruning, and synaptic reorganization [11, 12], among other alterations. Significant changes in the volume and shape of the hippocampal complex, a brain region that plays an important role in memory functions, are also observed during this developmental period [13–15].

Due to this plasticity, the adolescent brain seems to be especially vulnerable to the neurotoxic effects of alcohol. In fact, alcohol-related performance deficits in tasks assessing cognitive processes, such as attention, memory, and executive functions, in the not-yet-adult brain are more evident during adolescence [16, 17] and become more pronounced with a BD pattern of consumption [12, 18].

The intermittence between BD episodes seems to be the most important factor involved, as the repeated alternation between intoxication and withdrawal is particularly deleterious for the brain, due to the excitotoxic cell death it provokes [19, 20]. Thus, it has been demonstrated that BD episodes can be more harmful for the brain than an equivalent amount of alcohol without withdrawal episodes [20, 21].

Therefore, the BD adolescent population constitutes a cohort at risk of brain damage, and any disruptive effects of alcohol on learning and memory abilities in

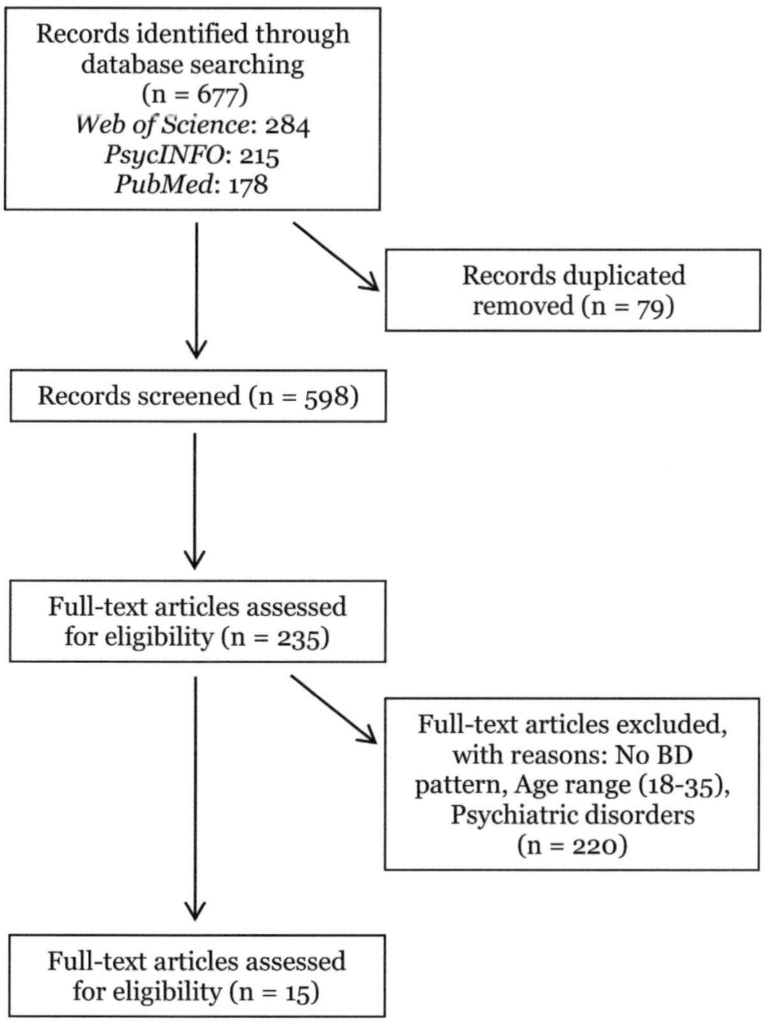

Figure 2.
Preferred reporting items for systematic reviews and meta-analyses (PRISMA) flow diagram showing how articles were selected for review.

this age group could have a particularly deep impact and last through to adulthood. Moreover, females would seem to be more vulnerable to these detrimental effects of alcohol [22].

In the following sections, the main insights provided by studies performed by our group and other researchers about the effects of BD on learning and memory performance will be discussed. We focus on the types of memory that are most damaged by alcohol: immediate visual memory (IVM) and working memory (WM). One distinctive contribution of this chapter is to evaluate, together, the impact of an acute BD episode and the sample's history of consumption on learning and memory performance, as well as the possible gender differences at play.

For this review, we conducted a literature search of three databases: *Web of Science*, *PsycINFO*, and *PubMed*. The following combination of key terms was used: binge/heavy/social OR adolescent/young OR blood alcohol OR immediate/working/ memory OR alcohol/ethanol OR cognitive AND acute alcohol. These keywords were examined in the "title" section for *Web of Science* and *PsycINFO* and "title/abstract" sections for *PubMed*. We considered studies published in English since 2000 (1 January 2000–30 November 2018) in humans. The total number of studies identified through the initial database searching was 677 (*Web of Science*, 284 records; *PsycINFO*, 215 records; *PubMed*, 178 records). Duplicated records were removed, and other articles were excluded using strict exclusion criteria: no BD pattern, out of age range (18–35 years old), psychiatric disorders, and other criteria described in the "methods" section. Eventually, 15 full-text articles were included in this review (see **Figure 2** and **Table 1**). This review is limited by the publication bias (databases not included), procedure of selection bias, and unavailable data.

2. Methods

2.1 Subjects

The experimental subjects in our studies (e.g., [23, 24]) were adolescent university students, who filled in a self-report questionnaire about consumption of drugs, frequency and level of alcohol consumption, hours and quality of sleep, and physical and psychological health. They were recruited based on strict inclusion and exclusion criteria. The inclusion criteria used were 18–19 years old, a healthy body mass index (between 20 and 25), and good health (without major medical problems). The subjects had to be refrainers (or very occasional alcohol consumers) or binge drinkers. The exclusion criteria were as follows: on medication; a history of mental disorders (diagnosed by a health professional according to DSM criteria); an irregular sleep pattern (non-restorative sleep and/or irregular schedule); having consumed, albeit sporadically, any drug (apart from alcohol) or having a history of substance abuse, including caffeine (our criterion: ≤2 stimulant drinks/day), tobacco (our criterion: ≤10 cigarettes/day), and alcohol (except for the BD consumption pattern); and having first-degree relatives with a history of alcoholism.

Other studies reviewed in this chapter included adolescents and young adults (18–35 years old) selected by similar or less restrictive inclusion/exclusion criteria, considering the alcohol use of subjects (history of problems due to alcohol use) and a history of mental health treatment (e.g., [25]).

2.2 Gender

Gender differences in the effects of alcohol have been reported, supporting the view that the brains of male and female adolescents are differentially affected by alcohol use [22]. There is evidence suggesting that female adolescents are more vulnerable to the neurotoxic effects of alcohol on cognition [22, 26, 27], since the cognitive tolerance effect of alcohol on IVM develops in BD women but not in BD men [24]. Other authors have found that men generally report lower sensitivity to alcohol (individuals need more alcohol to experience the same sensations or impairments) than women, and reactivity to alcohol-related cues is more pronounced in male than in female binge drinkers (e.g., [11]). These results might at least partially explain why men typically show a higher prevalence of alcohol consumption than women. However, in Spain at least, the incidence of alcohol consumption in 14–18-year-old adolescents is higher among females than males [4], while the BD pattern during adolescence is similar in 14–16-year-old adolescents and is more common among men than women in the age range of 17–18 years [4].

Gender differences in WM have also been reported in healthy young subjects, showing an advantage in this memory among males, with females exhibiting disadvantages manifested by a small effect size in both verbal and visuospatial WM [28]. This male advantage could be due to the activating effects of testosterone [29], though age and specific task modulate the magnitude and direction of the effects (e.g., [28, 30]). However, there are reviews in literature that explore the history of BD consumption but not the acute effects it exerts and which does not support the existence of gender differences in the effects of alcohol on this type of memory (e.g., [31]).

In the light of these data, it would seem crucial to consider (a) including both sexes, men and women, in any studies carried out and (b) evaluating potential gender differences in the relationship between BD and memory in adolescents and young adults.

2.3 Pattern alcohol consumption

Selected subjects were invited to participate in our studies if they reported refraining from alcohol consumption (or having indulged in very sporadic consumption) or a history of alcohol use classified as a BD pattern according to the NIAAA criteria for Spain (see [12]). Subsequently, the participants were classified as fulfilling a BD pattern if they had drunk six or more standard drink units (SDU) in the case of men or five or more SDU in the case of women on a minimum of two or three occasions per month throughout the 12 months prior to the survey. In Spain a SDU = 10 g of alcohol of distilled spirits (alcohol content ≥40% vol.). It is important to clarify that a stable BD pattern maintained over the time (12 months in the case of our studies) is a crucial criterion, because repeated alternation between intoxication and abstinence has been shown to be particularly harmful to the developing brain [19, 20]. Participants were classified as refrainers if they had never consumed alcoholic beverages or had drunk very sporadically (<1 SDU on <3 occasions per year, for example, 250 ml of beer, per occasion) since the onset of their alcohol use.

Therefore, in the studies reviewed in this chapter, including ours:

A. The experimental subjects were nondependent individuals indulging in alcohol use, usually evaluated by the Alcohol Use Disorders Identification Test (AUDIT) or others, such as the brief Michigan Alcoholism Screening test (e.g., [25]).

B. A very noticeable factor is the variability both in the samples' history (refrainers, habitual consumers, binge drinkers, light binge drinkers, etc.) and in the acute administration of alcohol that leads to a BAC of 0.8 g/L (see

Table 1 "sample's history of consumption" and "cognitive performance—with (BAC)—" entries for details).

C. Depending on the study, performance in the memory task was registered as either rising or declining BACs.

D. Taking into account the scarcity of studies evaluating acute alcohol consumption in adolescent and young adult refrainers or occasional consumers (e.g., [23]), the present chapter provides unique insights into this field of research.

2.4 Memory tests

In our studies, the third edition of the Wechsler Memory Scale (WMS-III; version adapted for the Spanish population) [32] was used to assess IVM and WM. The IVM subscales require the respondent to recognize faces and remember scenes, while the WM subscales require the respondent to put letter-number sets in order and to reproduce visual-spatial sequences. The literature reports a poorer performance in these types of memory under the acute effects of alcohol (e.g., [24, 33]) and especially in WM associated with a stable BD maintained in time (e.g., [34]).

Other scales used for the evaluation of these or similar types of memory are:

- The Cambridge Neuropsychological Test Automated Battery (CANTAB) for evaluating spatial recognition memory. The CANTAB is a computer-based cognitive assessment system consisting of a battery of neuropsychological tests, administered to subjects using a touch screen computer. This battery evaluates several areas of cognitive function using nonverbal stimuli in the majority of its tests, including the pattern recognition memory, a test of visual recognition memory in a two-choice forced discrimination paradigm.

- The Immediate Post-Concussion Assessment and Cognitive Testing (ImPACT) for evaluating long- and short-term memory, working memory, and declarative memory. The ImPACT is a computer-based program for assessing neurocognitive function and concussion symptoms. This neurocognitive test battery consists of several modules for evaluating attentional processes, verbal recognition memory, visual working memory, visual processing speed, reaction time, and numerical sequencing ability.

- The Wechsler Adult Intelligence Scale (WAIS-R) with the digit symbol substitution test (DSST) for evaluating short-term memory. The WAIS-R (revised form of the WAIS, a test designed to measure intelligence and cognitive ability in adults and older adolescents) consisted of six verbal and five performance subtests, including the DSST. This subtest (DSST-WAIS-R) consists of digit-symbol pairs followed by a list of digits; under each digit the subject must write down the corresponding symbol as fast as possible within the allowed time.

Obviously, the use of different tests/batteries for evaluating memory contributes to the heterogeneity of results in this field of research.

2.5 Procedure

In our procedure, all participants signed an informed consent and a data confidentiality agreement on arrival at the laboratory. BAC was measured in all subjects with an alcoholmeter to ensure that they had not previously drunk alcohol on the day in question, and the alcohol use of the BD adolescent subjects was assessed using the AUDIT test (none of the subjects was assessed as alcohol-dependent). Next, refrainers and binge drinkers drank 330 ml of lime- or orange-flavored refreshment (control groups), and binge drinkers' drank a high dose of alcohol. Alcohol was administered in a fixed dose of 120 ml (38.4 g) consisting of vodka mixed with the abovementioned refreshment for both genders or in function of their body weight (0.9 g alcohol/kg body weight in men and 0.8 g alcohol/kg body weight in women). The subjects were instructed to consume their drink within a period of 20 min. After finishing the drink, all subjects rinsed their mouths with water, and BAC was repeatedly measured every 5 min throughout the waiting period, until it reached a peak (approximately 20 min after consuming the drink). This peak of BAC was considered the value with which to classify the participants into the different experimental groups. The subjects performed the IVM and WM tests, while BAC was descendent. BAC was measured once again at the beginning of the tests, between the tests and at the end of the experiment. The BACs registered for the male and female subjects (separately or together) in the different experimental groups were:

A. 0.0 g/L, in refrainers men (n = 17) and women (n = 24) or BD men (n = 23) and women (n = 27). These are control groups receiving a nonalcoholic drink.

B. 0.33 g/L, in refrainers men (n = 17) or BD men (n = 22).

C. 0.38 g/L, in refrainers men (n = 11) and women (n = 11) or BD men (n = 11) and women (n = 11).

D. 0.5 g/L, in refrainers (n = 18) or BD women (n = 24).

E. 0.3–0.5 g/L (mean = 0.4 g/L), in BD men (n = 12) and women (n = 12).

F. 0.54–1.1 g/L (mean = 0.8 g/L), in BD men (n = 14) and women (n = 24).

(Note: The A, B, C, and D experimental groups belong to Ref. 23; and the A, E, and F experimental groups belong to Ref. 24).

All tests were performed between 4:00 pm and 8:00 pm, and the subjects that received alcohol remained on the premises until their alcohol concentration dropped to legal limits for driving (<0.3 g/L).

Similar procedures were applied in the other reviewed studies, where cognitive performance—with (BAC)—was evaluated after alcohol intake administered in fixed doses or according to body weight. Participants also abstained from alcohol for at least 12 h prior to the experiment, as well as drinking coffee or tea on the mornings prior to the experiment, and were instructed to eat a low-fat breakfast and lunch on the day on which tests were performed (e.g., [35]).

3. Results

The main findings obtained in our experimental investigations and those of other groups are summarized in **Table 1**. The effects of acute alcohol consumption—one BD episode with different BACs—on different types of memory are reviewed.

A total number of 15 studies are summarized. Only three of them included adolescent male and females (18–20 years old) [23, 24, 33]; the participants in the rest of the studies were in the 18–35-year-old group, without studies comparing adolescents and young adults.

The sample's history of consumption encompasses a range from refrainers to heavy binge drinkers, including habitual consumers/moderate drinkers and light binge drinkers. This variability in the samples of the reviewed studies gives us a more specific view of the acute effects of alcohol in different types of consumers and not only in binge drinkers.

In general, the results obtained in the evaluated memory tasks confirm the deleterious effects of alcohol use. Significant impairments were observed in spatial recognition memory, WM, associative learning, word fragment completion, free recall, long-term memory, short-term memory, and IVM. However, an absence of effects has also been observed with respect to some of these memories, such as visual memory, short-term memory, WM, and IVM. It is possible that the impairing effects observed are conditioned by BAC (ascendant BAC, BAC peak, descendant BAC) in the case of some types of memory. Thus, in studies in which there were

Sample	***Sample's history of consumption***	***Memory/Test***	***Cognitive performance -with (BAC)-***	***Ref.***
N = 50 (18-34 years old) Men/Women	BD (12-45 SDU/week)	↓ Spatial recognition memory (CANTAB)	BD (0.59-0.52 g/L) < Placebo	[35]
N = 41 (≥ 18 years old) Men	BD (≥ 8 SDU /week) / Light BD (< 8 SDU /week)	↓ WM (Random Object Span Task)	BD and Light BD (0.8 g/L) < Placebo	[36]
		↓ Associative learning	Light BD (0.8 g/L) < Placebo	
N = 72 (19-25 years old) Men/Women	Habitual consumers (1.11 ml ethanol/kg weight and 1.2 occasions/week)	↓ WM (Sternberg Memory Scanning task)	Habitual consumers (ascendant BAC 0.68-0.86 g/L) < Placebo	[37]
		= WM (Sternberg Memory Scanning task)	Habitual consumers (descendant BAC 0.86-0.64 g/L) = Placebo	
N = 69 (21-29 years old) Men	Habitual consumers (3.9 SDU and 2.3 occasions/week)	↓ Associative learning	Habitual consumers (0.8 g/L) < Placebo	[38]
		↓ Word fragment completion	Habitual consumers (0.3 g/L) < Placebo	
		↓ Free recall	Habitual consumers (0.3 g/L) < Placebo	
		= Visual memory (Picture recognition)	Habitual consumers (0.8 g/L) = Placebo	

N = 20 (21,8 mean years old) Men	--	↓ Long-term memory (ImPACT)	Alcohol consumers (ascendant BAC: 0.81-0.93 g/L) < Placebo	[39]
		↓ Long-term visual memory (ImPACT)	Alcohol consumers (ascendant BAC: 0,81-0.93 g/L) < Placebo	
		↓ Short-term memory (ImPACT)	Alcohol consumers (ascendant BAC: 0.81-0.93 g/L) < Placebo	
		↓ WM (ImPACT)	Alcohol consumers (ascendant BAC: 0.81-0.93 g/L) < Placebo	
		↓ Declarative memory (ImPACT)	Alcohol consumers (ascendant BAC: 0.81-0.93 g/L) < Placebo	
		= WM (ImPACT)	Alcohol consumers (descendant BAC 0.86-0.79 g/L) = Placebo	
		= Short-term memory (ImPACT)	Alcohol consumers (descendant BAC 0.86-0.79 g/L) = Placebo	
N = 72 (21-35 years old) Men/Women	BD (≥ 10 SDU and 1.5 occasions/week) / Light BD (< 6 SDU /week)	↓ Short-term memory (DSST-WAIS-R)	BD (0.92 g/L) < Placebo Light BD (0.82 g/L) < Placebo	[40]
		= Short-term memory (DSST-WAIS-R)	BD (0.42 g/L) = Placebo Light BD (0.36 g/L) = Placebo BD = Light BD	
N = 72 (21-30 years old) Men/Women	BD (2-24 SDU /week)	↓ WM	BD (0.9 g/L) < Placebo	[41]
N = 27 (21-35 years old) Men/Women	Habitual consumers (5 SDU /week)	= Short-term memory (DSST-WAIS-R)	Acute consumers of 0.8 g alcohol/kg weight = Placebo	[42]
N = 10 (19-29 years old) Men/Women	Habitual consumers (12-30 SDU /month)	= Visual WM [43]	Habitual consumers (0.6 g/L) = Placebo	[44]
N = 32 (18-30 years old) Men	Habitual consumers (31.8-36.3 SDU /week)	= WM (Spatial Span)	Habitual consumers (0.73 g/L) = Placebo	[45]

		= WM (Baddeley's Reasoning task)	Habitual consumers (0.73 g/L) = Placebo	
N = 91 (18-20 years old) Men/Women	--	↓ WM (Trail Making Test- Trail B)	Alcohol consumers (0.84 g/L) < Placebo	[33]
N = 19 (18-35 years old) Men	Habitual consumers (≥ 4 SDU and 2 occasions/month)	↓ Short-term memory (DSST-WAIS-R)	Placebo > habitual consumers (0.78 g/L)	[46]
N = 75 (21-35 years old) Men/women	Moderate drinkers / Heavy drinkers	= WM (Wais-III and IV)	Moderate-Heavy drinkers (0.63 g/L) = Moderate-Heavy drinkers (0.0 g/L)	[25]
		= WM (Trail Making Test- Trail A-B)	Moderate-Heavy drinkers (0.63 g/L) = Moderate-Heavy drinkers (0.0 g/L)	
N = 79 (18-19 years old) Men	Refrainers / BD (≥ 6 SDU and ≥ 20ccasions/ month)	= Immediate visual memory (Wechsler-III)	Refrainers (0.0 g/L) = Refrainers (0.33 g/L) = BD (0.0 g/L) = BD (0.33 g/L)	[23]
		= WM (Wechsler-III)	Refrainers (0.0 g/L) = Refrainers (0.33 g/L) = BD (0.0 g/L) = BD (0.33 g/L)	
N = 93 (18-19 years old) Women	Refrainers / BD (≥ 5 SDU and ≥ 20ccasions/ month)	↓ Immediate visual memory (Wechsler-III)	Refrainers (0,5 g/L) < Refrainers (0.0 g/L)	[23]
			BD (0.0 g/L) < Refrainers (0.0 g/L)	
			Refrainers (0.5 g/L) < BD (0.5 g/L)	
		= WM (Wechsler-III)	Refrainers (0.0 g/L) = Refrainers (0.5 g/L) = BD (0.0 g/L) = BD (0.5 g/L)	

N = 136 (18-19 years old) Men/Women	Refrainers / BD (Men ≥ 6 SDU, women ≥ 5 SDU; and ≥ 2occasions/ month)	↓ Immediate visual memory (Wechsler-III)	Men BD (0.38 g/L) < Men BD (0.0 g/L)	[23]
			Women Refrainers (0.38 g/L) < Women Refrainers (0.0 g/L)	
		= WM (Wechsler-III)	Refrainers (0.0 g/L) = Refrainers (0.38 g/L) = BD (0.0 g/L) = BD (0.38 g/L)	
N = 154 (18-19 years old) Men/Women	Refrainers / BD (Men ≥ 6 SDU, women ≥ 5 SDU; and ≥ 2occasions/ month)	↓ Immediate visual memory (Wechsler-III)	BD (0.4 g/L) < Refrainers (0.0 g/L)	[24]
			BD (0.8 g/L) < BD (0.0 g/L) = Refrainers (0.0 g/L)	
		↓ WM (Wechsler-III)	BD (0.8 g/L) < BD (0.4 g/L) = BD (0.0 g/L) = Refrainers (0.0 g/L)	

Table 1.
Effects of acute alcohol consumption (one BD episode with different BACs) on memory in the studies carried out in this field [37, 39, 42, 43 and 46].

ascendant and descendant BACs, impairment was reported in long-term memory, short-term memory, and WM declarative memory with ascendant BAC but not with descendant BAC.

Finally, the values for cognitive performance—with (BAC)—in **Table 1** show the absence of effects or impairing effects in every sample, including for BAC of 0.0 g/L (refrainers and binge drinkers consuming refreshment/placebo). For example, in Vinader-Caerols et al. [23], male IVM performance was refrainers (0.0 g/L) = refrainers (0.33 g/L) = BD (0.0 g/L) = BD (0.33 g/L) and women's performance was BD (0.0 g/L) < refrainers (0.0 g/L).

4. Discussion

The key findings of this review will now be discussed. Among the types of memory reviewed, word fragment completion, free recall, and IVM appear to be the most sensitive to the effects of acute alcohol, as they are affected by moderate doses of alcohol (BAC = 0.3–0.38 g/L) in adolescents and young adults (e.g., [23, 38]). However, higher doses of alcohol (BAC levels of BD, i.e., around 0.8 g/L) are necessary for a significant impairment in other memories, such as WM (e.g., [24]) and short-term memory (e.g., [40]). A plausible explanation for the lack of effects reported with BACs under 0.8 g/L (e.g., [23, 25, 40, 44, 45]) is that the brain of binge drinkers employs compensatory mechanisms in additional brain areas to perform the tasks adequately and that these resources are undermined at higher BACs (e.g., [24, 33, 36, 40, 41]).

In contrast to the present review, others have attempted to provide an overview of affected (and unaffected) neuropsychological functions in adolescents and young binge drinkers, without evaluating the acute effects of alcohol and considering only the subjects' history of BD (e.g., [31]). However, the interaction between a BD history of consumption and the effects of acute alcohol exposure on learning and memory needs to be studied, as some long-term effects of repeated alcohol exposure in adolescents (such as alcohol tolerance or damaged cognitive abilities) are observed more readily—if at all—following an acute dose of alcohol [23].

It is known that tolerance can develop early in adolescents and young adults without alcohol use disorder [47, 48]. Considering the scarcity of studies that have evaluated the phenomenon of tolerance in healthy adolescents and the potential vulnerability of females to the neurotoxic effects of alcohol, we performed a study [23] in which we observed that binge drinkers performed better in IVM than refrainers when given alcohol (showing the development of alcohol tolerance) and binge drinkers performed worse than refrainers after consuming a nonalcoholic control drink (as their memory would have been damaged). Thus, adolescent women are more vulnerable to the neurotoxic effects of alcohol than men, because the cognitive tolerance effect of alcohol on IVM develops in BD women but not in BD men. The phenomenon of women beginning to drink earlier and progressing more rapidly than men from drinking onset to problematic drinking, known as the "telescoping effect" [49–51], would explain why adolescent women develop cognitive tolerance earlier than men.

Although men and women have been included in some of the reviewed studies, only ours [23, 24] were carried out in order to specifically evaluate these gender differences in adolescents. In our second study [24], although the tolerance phenomenon was not evaluated (because refrainers did not consume an acute dose of alcohol), no gender differences were detected in IVM and WM performance with BAC > 0.5 mg/L. We suspect that an increased BAC overrides these cognitive differences between men and women. At the same time, the BAC is dependent on several factors such as rates of absorption, distribution, and elimination, as well as gender, body mass and composition, food effects, and type of alcohol. Therefore, careful extrapolation and interpretation of the BAC is needed [52].

The findings of the present review would be bolstered with a tighter control of factors that contribute to heterogeneity of results, such as:

- Not taking into account the gender factor. The inclusion of men and women in study samples is more representative of the population.

- Variability in the sample's history of consumption, which can encompass a wide range (refrainers, habitual consumers/moderate drinkers, light binge drinkers, heavy binge drinkers, etc.).

- The use of different tests/batteries for evaluating similar memories (e.g., CANTAB, ImPACT, WAIS-R).

- The registration of performance in ascendant/descendant BACs. For example, more deleterious effects are observed in ascendant BAC versus descendant BAC. Most of the studies either they evaluate memory performance in descendant BAC or they do not specify whether the BAC is ascendant or descendant.

- Variability in the age ranges in the studies. This variability (see **Table 1**), without a neat separation between adolescents and young adults, does not allow to properly compare these periods in order to find potential differences. Actually, there are not studies directly evaluating possible differences in the effects of acute BD on memory, comparing adolescents and young adults.

Several studies, using different paradigms (e.g., Stroop task, Go/No-Go task), have also shown that BD during adolescence is associated with poor inhibitory control (e.g., [7, 53]). Inhibitory control processes are developing during adolescence and youth, and a poor inhibitory function may predispose the individual to alcohol misuse [53]. Thus, impaired inhibitory control has been related to increased loss of control over drinking (i.e., a greater number of drinks per episode) [7], and this impairment seems to be related to the severity of alcohol-related problems [54, 55]. Likewise, acute and binge alcohol drinking may impair the inhibitory control and compromise the ability to prevent or stop behavior related to alcohol use. Then, poor inhibitory control can be both the cause and the consequence of excessive alcohol use. Adolescence and young adulthood may be a particularly vulnerable period due to the following reasons: (a) the weak or immature inhibitory functioning typical of this stage may contribute to the inability of the individual to control alcohol use and (b) alcohol consumption per se may alter or interrupt the proper development of inhibitory control leading to a reduced ability to regulate alcohol intake [53]. Therefore, inhibitory control training is a potential effective component of a comprehensive protocol for intervention strategies focused on this at-risk group of young adults who continue a BD trajectory into adulthood. Interventions targeting binge-drinking behavior should aim to inhibitory control training.

Increasing the knowledge about the effects of BD alcohol consumption pattern on memory and other executive functions in adolescents and young adults is also instrumental to designing programs and policy to reduce the impact of drinking in this highly vulnerable population in order to diminish the likelihood of participation in risky behaviors.

5. Conclusions

After reviewing the literature concerning the effects of one BD episode (with different BACs) on learning and memory performance in adolescents and young adults, the following conclusions can be drawn:

- Alcohol BD has differential effects depending on the type of memory. For example, IVM is more sensitive than other memories to the neurotoxic effects of acute doses of alcohol in adolescents and young adults with a BD history (IVM is affected by a moderate BAC, while WM score is undermined only by BAC levels of BD).

- BAC is an important factor to take into account when evaluating the acute effects of BD alcohol on memory performance in this type of studies.

- Women are more vulnerable to some of the detrimental effects of alcohol than men are. For example, an effect of cognitive alcohol tolerance on IVM has been observed in women but not in men. These gender differences emphasize the need to include females in studies when investigating the neurotoxic effects of alcohol in adolescents and youths.

- Further research, particularly longitudinal studies, is necessary in order to confirm the abovementioned findings and to consolidate these conclusions.

In relation to the inhibitory control in binge drinkers, taking into account the scarcity of studies evaluating inhibitory control training on alcohol consumption (e.g., [56–58]) and the lack of them evaluating this kind of training on BD, future research should investigate long-term implementation of inhibitory control training, emphasizing the importance of this training as part of the intervention strategies focused on this at-risk group.

Acknowledgements

The authors wish to thank the "Generalitat Valenciana" [PROMETEO-II/2015/020] and the "Universitat de València" [UV-INV_AE18-779336] for the funding part of the work reviewed herein. They also wish to thank Mr. Brian Normanly for his editorial assistance.

Conflict of interest

The authors have no conflict of interest to declare.

Author details

Concepción Vinader-Caerols* and Santiago Monleón
Department of Psychobiology, University of Valencia, Valencia, Spain

*Address all correspondence to: concepcion.vinader@uv.es

References

[1] Hibell B, Guttormsson U, Ahlström S, Balakireva O, Bjarnason T, Kokkevi A, Kraus L. Substance use among students in 35 European Countries (The 2007 European School Survey Project on Alcohol and other Drugs, ESPAD, Report). Stockholm: The European Monitoring Center for Drugs and Drug Addiction; 2007

[2] Chavez PR, Nelson DE, Naimi TS, Brewer RD. Impact of a new gender-specific definition for binge drinking on prevalence estimates for women. American Journal of Preventive Medicine. 2011;**40**:468-471

[3] National Institute of Alcohol Abuse and Alcoholism. NIAAA council approves definition of binge drinking. NIAAA Newsletter. 2004;**3**:3

[4] Observatorio Español sobre Drogas (OED). Encuesta Escolar sobre Uso de Drogas en Estudiantes de Enseñanzas Secundarias (ESTUDES) 2014–2015. Madrid: Ministerio de Sanidad, Servicios Sociales e Igualdad; 2016

[5] Gil-Hernandez S, Garcia-Moreno LM. Executive performance and dysexecutive symptoms in binge drinking adolescents. Alcohol. 2016;**51**: 79-87. DOI: 10.1016/j.alcohol. 2016.01.003

[6] Poulton A, Mackenzie C, Harrington K, Borg S, Hester R. Cognitive control over immediate reward in binge alcohol drinkers. Alcoholism, Clinical and Experimental Research. 2016;**40**:429-437. DOI: 10.1111/acer.12968

[7] Carbia C, Corral M, Doallo S, Caamaño-Isorna F. The dual-process model in young adults with a consistent binge drinking trajectory into adulthood. Drug and Alcohol Dependence. 2018;**186**:113-119. DOI: 10.1016/j.drugalcdep.2018.01.023

[8] Herman AM, Critchley HD, Duka T. Binge drinking is associated with attenuated frontal and parietal activation during successful response inhibition in fearful context. The European Journal of Neuroscience. 2018: 1-14. DOI: 10.1111/ejn.14108

[9] Cohen-Gilbert JE, Nickerson LD, Sneider JT, Oot EN, Seraikas AM, Rohan ML, et al. College binge drinking associated with decreased frontal activation to negative emotional distractors during inhibitory control. Frontiers in Psychology. 2017;**8**:1650. DOI: 10.3389/fpsyg.2017.01650

[10] Blakemore SJ. The social brain in adolescence. Nature Reviews. Neuroscience. 2008;**9**:267-277

[11] Petit G, Kornreich C, Verbanck P, Campanella S. Gender differences in reactivity to alcohol cues in binge drinkers: A preliminary assessment of event-related potentials. Psychiatry Research. 2013;**209**:494-503. DOI: 10.1016/j.psychres.2013.04.005

[12] López-Caneda E, Mota N, Crego A, Velasquez T, Corral M, Rodríguez Holguín S, et al. Neurocognitive anomalies associated with the binge drinking pattern of alcohol consumption in adolescents and young people: A review. Adicciones. 2014;**26**:334-359. DOI: 10.20882/adicciones.39

[13] Gogtay N, Nugent TF 3rd, Herman DH, Ordonez A, Greenstein D, Hayashi KM, et al. Dynamic mapping of normal human hippocampal development. Hippocampus. 2006;**16**: 664-672. DOI: 10.1002/hipo.20193

[14] DeMaster D, Pathman T, Lee JK, Ghetti S. Structural development of the hippocampus and episodic memory: Developmental differences along the anterior/posterior axis. Cerebral Cortex.

2014;**24**:3036-3045. DOI: 10.1093/cercor/bht160

[15] Krogsrud SK, Tamnes CK, Fjell AM, Amlien I, Grydeland H, Sulutvedt U, et al. Development of hippocampal subfield volumes from 4 to 22 years. Human Brain Mapping. 2014;**35**: 5646-5657. DOI: 10.1002/hbm.22576

[16] Crean R, Vandewater S, Katner S, Huitron-Resendiz S, Taffe M. Chronic alcohol consumption impairs visuo-spatial associative memory in periadolescent rhesus monkeys. Drug and Alcohol Dependence. 2010;**114**:31-40. DOI: 10.1016/j.drugalcdep.2010.09.002

[17] Risher ML, Fleming RL, Boutros N, Semenova S, Wilson WA, Levin ED, et al. Long-term effects of chronic intermittent ethanol exposure in adolescent and adult rats: Radial-arm maze performance and operant food reinforced responding. PLoS One. 2013; **13, 8**(5):e62940. DOI: 10.1371/journal.pone.0062940

[18] Peeters M, Vollebergh WA, Wiers RW, Field M. Psychological changes and cognitive impairments in adolescent heavy drinkers. Alcohol and Alcoholism. 2014;**49**:182-186. DOI: 10.1093/alcalc/agt162

[19] Maurage P, Joassin F, Speth A, Modave J, Philippot P, Campanella S. Cerebral effects of binge drinking: Respective influences of global alcohol intake and consumption pattern. Clinical Neurophysiology. 2012;**123**: 892-901. DOI: 10.1016/j.clinph.2011.09.018

[20] Petit G, Maurage P, Kornreich C, Verbanck P, Campanella S. Binge drinking in adolescents: A review of neurophysiological and neuroimaging research. Alcohol and Alcoholism. 2014; **49**:198-206. DOI: 10.1093/alcalc/agt172

[21] Duka T, Gentry J, Malcolm R, Ripley TL, Borlikova G, Stephens DN, et al. Consequences of multiple withdrawals from alcohol. Alcoholism, Clinical and Experimental Research. 2004;**280**:233-246. DOI: 10.1097/01.ALC.0000113780.41701.81

[22] Alfonso-Loeches S, Pascual M, Guerri C. Gender differences in alcohol-induced neurotoxicity and brain damage. Toxicology. 2013;**311**:27-34. DOI: 10.1016/j.tox.2013.03.001

[23] Vinader-Caerols C, Talk A, Montañés A, Duque A, Monleón S. Differential effects of alcohol on memory performance in adolescent men and women with binge drinking history. Alcohol and Alcoholism. 2017;**52**: 610-616. DOI: 10.1093/alcalc/agx040

[24] Vinader-Caerols C, Duque A, Montañés A, Monleón S. Blood alcohol concentration-related lower performance in immediate visual memory and working memory in adolescent binge drinkers. Frontiers in Psychology. 2017;**8**:1720. DOI: 10.3389/fpsyg.2017.01720

[25] Spinola S, Maisto SA, White CN, Huddleson T. Effects of acute alcohol intoxication on executive functions controlling self-regulated behavior. Alcohol. 2017;**61**:1-8. DOI: 10.1016/j.alcohol.2017.02.177

[26] Caldwell LC, Schweinsburg AD, Nagel BJ, Barlett VC, Brown SA, Tapert SF. Gender and adolescent alcohol use disorders on BOLD (blood oxygen level dependent) response to spatial working memory. Alcohol and Alcoholism. 2005;**40**:194-200. DOI: 10.1093/alcalc/agh134

[27] Squeglia LM, Schweinsburg AD, Pulido C, Tapert SF. Adolescent binge drinking linked to abnormal spatial working memory brain activation: Differential gender effects. Alcoholism, Clinical and Experimental Research. 2011;**35**:1831-1841. DOI: 10.1111/j.1530-0277.2011.01527.x

[28] Zilles D, Lewandowski M, Vieker H, Henseler I, Diekhof E, Melcher T, et al. Gender differences in verbal and visuospatial working memory performance and networks. Neuropsychobiology. 2016;**73**:52-63. DOI: 10.1159/000443174

[29] Janowsky JS, Chavez B, Orwoll E. Sex steroids modify working memory. Journal of Cognitive Neuroscience. 2000;**12**:407-414. DOI: 10.1162/089892900562228

[30] Voyer D, Voyer SD, Saint-Aubin J. Sex differences in visual-spatial working memory: A meta-analysis. Psychonomic Bulletin & Review. 2017;**24**:307-334. DOI: 10.3758/s13423-016-1085-7

[31] Carbia C, López-Caneda E, Corral M, Cadaveira F. A systematic review of neuropsychological studies involving young binge drinkers. Neuroscience and Biobehavioral Reviews. 2018;**90**:332-349. DOI: 10.1016/j.neubiorev.2018.04.013

[32] Wechsler D. Wechsler Adult Intelligence Scale-III. San Antonio, EEUU: The Psychological Corporation; 2004

[33] Day AM, Celio MA, Lisman SA, Johansen GE, Spear LP. Acute and chronic effects of alcohol on trail making test performance among underage drinkers in a field setting. Journal of Studies on Alcohol and Drugs. 2013;**74**:635-641. DOI: 10.15288/jsad.2013.74.635

[34] Carbia C, Cadaveira F, López-Caneda E, Caamaño-Isorna F, Rodríguez Holguín S, Corral M. Working memory over a six-year period in young binge drinkers. Alcohol. 2017; **61**:17-23. DOI: 10.1016/j.alcohol.2017.01.013

[35] Weissenborn R, Duka T. Acute alcohol effects on cognitive function in social drinkers: Their relationship to drinking habits. Psychopharmacology. 2003;**165**:306-312

[36] Pihl RO, Paylan SS, Gentes-Hawn A, Hoaken PN. Alcohol affects executive cognitive functioning differentially on the ascending versus descending limb of the blood alcohol concentration curve. Alcoholism, Clinical and Experimental Research. 2003;**27**:773-779

[37] Grattan-Miscio KE, Vogel-Sprott M. Effects of alcohol and performance incentives on immediate working memory. Psychopharmacology. 2005; **181**:188-196. DOI: 10.1007/s00213-005-2226-2

[38] Söderlund H, Parker ES, Schwartz BL, Tulving E. Memory encoding and retrieval on the ascending and descending limbs of the blood alcohol concentration curve. Psychopharmacology. 2005;**182**:305-317. DOI: 10.1007/ s00213-005-0096-2

[39] Schweizer TA, Vogel-Sprott M, Danckert J, Roy EA, Skakum A, Broderick CE. Neuropsychological profile of acute alcohol intoxication during ascending and descending blood alcohol concentrations. Neuropsychopharmacology. 2006;**31**: 1301-1309. DOI: 10.1038/sj.npp.1300941

[40] Brumback T, Cao D, King A. Effects of alcohol on psychomotor performance and perceived impairment in heavy binge social drinkers. Drug and Alcohol Dependence. 2007;**91**:10-17. DOI: 10.1016/j.drugalcdep. 2007.04.013

[41] Saults JS, Cowan N, Sher KJ, Moreno MV. Differential effects of alcohol on working memory: Distinguishing multiple processes. Experimental and Clinical Psychopharmacology. 2007;**15**:576-587. DOI: 10.1037/1064-1297.15.6.576

[42] Holdstock L, de Wit H. Individual differences in responses to ethanol and

d-amphetamine: A within-subject study. Alcoholism, Clinical and Experimental Research. 2001;**25**:540-548. DOI: 10.1111/j.1530-0277.2001.tb02248.x

[43] Luck SJ, Vogel EK. The capacity of visual working memory for features and conjunctions. Nature. 1997;**390**:279-281. DOI: 10.1038/36846

[44] Paulus MP, Tapert SF, Pulido C, Schuckit MA. Alcohol attenuates load-related activation during a working memory task: Relation to level of response to alcohol. Alcoholism, Clinical and Experimental Research. 2006;**30**: 1363-1371. DOI: 10.1111/j.1530-0277.2006.00164.x

[45] Rose AK, Duka T. The influence of alcohol on basic motoric and cognitive disinhibition. Alcohol and Alcoholism. 2007;**42**:544-551. DOI: 10.1093/alcalc/agm073

[46] Cash C, Peacock A, Barrington H, Sinnett N, Bruno R. Detecting impairment: Sensitive cognitive measures of dose-related acute alcohol intoxication. Journal of Psychopharmacology. 2015;**29**:436-446. DOI: 10.1177/0269881115570080

[47] Saha TD, Chou SP, Grant BF. Toward an alcohol use disorder continuum using item response theory: Results from the National Epidemiologic Survey on alcohol and related conditions. Psychological Medicine. 2006;**36**:931-941. DOI: 10.1017/S003329170600746X

[48] Schuckit MA, Smith TL, Hesselbrock V, Bucholz KK, Bierut L, Edenberg H, et al. Clinical implications of tolerance to alcohol in nondependent young drinkers. The American Journal of Drug and Alcohol Abuse. 2008;**34**:133-149. DOI: 10.1080/00952990701877003

[49] Piazza NJ, Vrbka JL, Yeager RD. Telescoping of alcoholism in women alcoholics. The International Journal of the Addictions. 1989;**24**:19-28

[50] Johnson PB, Richter L, Kleber HD, McLellan AT, Carise D. Telescoping of drinking-related behaviors: Gender, racial/ethnic, and age comparisons. Substance Use & Misuse. 2005;**40**: 1139-1151. DOI: 10.1081/JA-200042281

[51] Sugarman DE, Demartini KS, Carey KB. Are women at greater risk? An examination of alcohol-related consequences and gender. The American Journal on Addictions. 2009;**18**:194-197. DOI: 10.1080/10550490902786991

[52] Perry PJ, Doroudgar S, Van Dyke P. Ethanol forensic toxicology. The Journal of the American Academy of Psychiatry and the Law. 2017;**45**:429-438

[53] López-Caneda E, Rodríguez Holguín S, Cadaveira F, Corral M, Doallo S. Impact of alcohol use on inhibitory control (and vice versa) during adolescence and young adulthood: A review. Alcohol and Alcoholism. 2014;**49**:173-181. DOI: 10.1093/alcalc/agt168

[54] Claus ED, Feldstein Ewing SW, Filbey FM, Hutchison KE. Behavioral control in alcohol use disorders: Relationships with severity. Journal of Studies on Alcohol and Drugs. 2013;**74**: 141-151

[55] Smith JL, Mattick RP, Jamadar SD, Iredale JM. Deficits in behavioural inhibition in substance abuse and addiction: A meta-analysis. Drug and Alcohol Dependence. 2014;**145**:1-33. DOI: 10.1016/j.drugalcdep.2014.08.009.

[56] Bowley C, Faricy C, Hegarty B, Johnstone S, Smith JL, Kelly P, et al. The effects of inhibitory control training on alcohol consumption, implicit alcohol-related cognitions and brain electrical activity. International Journal of Psychophysiology. 2013;**89**:342-348. DOI: 10.1016/j.ijpsycho.2013.04.011

[57] Di Lemma LCG, Field M. Cue avoidance training and inhibitory control training for the reduction of alcohol consumption: A comparison of effectiveness and investigation of their mechanisms of action. Psychopharmacology. 2017;**234**: 2489-2498. DOI: 10.1007/s00213-017-4639-0

[58] Jones A, McGrath E, Robinson E, Houben K, Nederkoorn C, Field M. A randomized controlled trial of inhibitory control training for the reduction of alcohol consumption in problem drinkers. Journal of Consulting and Clinical Psychology. 2018;**86**: 991-1004. DOI: 10.1037/ccp0000312

Chapter 5

Life Stress and Inhibitory Control Deficits: Teaching BrainWise as a Neurocognitive Intervention in Vulnerable Populations

Marilyn Welsh, Patricia Gorman Barry and Jared M. Greenberg

Abstract

The chapter describes inhibitory control in the context of broader and related constructs, executive function and self-regulation. We discuss the adaptive functions of inhibitory control, as well as evidence that life stress, such as poverty, maltreatment, homelessness, and mental illness, negatively impacts individuals' inhibitory control and overall self-regulation skills. Moreover, these stressors are known to disrupt the development and functioning of crucial brain systems underlying inhibitory control. Following this review, we discuss a critical thinking skills intervention, BrainWise, which is designed to teach inhibitory and self-regulation skills to children, youth and adults. We describe the implementation of the program, and review evidence for its effectiveness with various populations, including our recent study that demonstrated the success of BrainWise in teaching these skills to homeless men living in transitional housing. Finally, we describe our proposed future applications of this intervention to veterans suffering serious mental health challenges. Our overarching goals are to highlight the importance of inhibitory control and overall self-regulation, the vulnerability of these important skills to life stress, and the promise held by one neurocognitive intervention for improving inhibitory control in high-risk populations.

Keywords: inhibitory control, executive function, self-regulation, stress, poverty, homelessness, childhood maltreatment, mental illness, intervention, BrainWise, veterans

1. Introduction

Inhibitory control, as a key component of goal-directed executive function and overall self-regulation, has implications for a range of adaptive behaviors across development. Individual differences in this self-regulatory ability have implications for accomplishing important life tasks such as educational achievement, securing employment, and establishing successful relationships. Failures to achieve these milestones has enormous personal costs, as well as economic costs to society. The contributions to these individual differences are complex covariations and interactions between biological and environmental forces [1], as is true for the wide swath of psychological development. How we respond to these individual differences, particularly at the lower end of functioning, with an appreciation of malleable environmental factors and intervention will determine the degree to which we can optimize inhibitory control, benefiting both individuals and the larger society.

The purpose of this chapter is to describe the construct that is the topic of this volume, inhibitory control. We view inhibitory control within the larger contexts of self-regulation, emotion regulation, and executive functions, skills that are all required for adaptive functioning in our increasingly complex world. We will describe the impacts of environmental challenges and life stresses, such as poverty, maltreatment, homelessness, and mental illness on the development and expression of inhibitory control. In addition, we will discuss how the neural mechanisms underlying inhibitory control and related processes are particularly vulnerable to these stressors.

The critical role that inhibitory control plays in adaptive behavior in a wide range of contexts, and its vulnerability to both environmental and biological challenges, has stimulated a diversity of interventions for children, adolescents, and adults in recent years with varying results. We will focus our discussion on one intervention that involves teaching critical thinking skills to promote inhibitory control and overall self-regulation. The BrainWise program will be described in terms of its design and effectiveness in facilitating adaptive decision making and behavior, particularly in high-risk populations. Finally, we will describe the inhibitory control and self-regulatory deficits observed in veterans experiencing mental illness and/or homelessness and a planned application of the BrainWise intervention to this vulnerable population.

2. Importance of inhibitory control to adaptive behavior

2.1 Inhibitory control defined

Inhibitory control is the ability to withhold responses to both internal and external signals when such responses would be maladaptive either for immediate functioning or in service of a future goal. The more adaptive alternative response in these situations involves flexible, reflective "top down" mechanisms that operate to control the "bottom-up" arousal, emotion, and stress responses that are often present in our highly-charged daily activities [2]. Research demonstrates that the development of inhibitory control predicts school readiness and performance in young children [2], as well as a range of academic and cognitive skills [3, 4]. In adolescents and young adults, the inability to control behavior, particularly in affectively- and motivationally-charged contexts, is predicative of maladaptive risk taking [5]. Developmental disorders that have documented difficulties with inhibitory control include: autism [6, 7], ADHD [8, 9], and disruptive behavior disorders [10]. Difficulties with inhibition represent impediments to the normal trajectory of development in social–emotional and academic domains, potentially setting up the individual for struggles in adaptation throughout their lifetime.

Difficulties with inhibitory control may be manifested as maladaptive impulsivity in behavior and is described by Nigg [11] as taking two forms. One form of impulsivity that reflects a non-reflective, immediate reactions to stimuli (either internal thoughts or external events) is often called disinhibition. This can be seen when a 3-year-old overtly expresses a reaction to someone's appearance in embarrassing fashion, or when an individual with frontal lobe damage continues to make an incorrect decision despite consciously knowing these decisions are wrong. Disinhibition may be a consequence of the life stresses that we will discuss in this chapter, such as extreme trauma or mental illness, particularly when these involve possible brain damage. The second type of impulsivity involves a motivated preference for an immediate reward over a delayed reward, even if the latter is bigger, better, and ultimately more rewarding [12]. Individual differences in inhibitory control are found in the typically-functioning population, mediated by particular brain regions, and appear to reflect temperamental differences in effortful control [13]. However, this propensity to seek out immediate rewards, even when ultimately maladaptive, also may be impacted by the stressors of poverty, trauma, homelessness, and mental illness, either through learning from one's environment, through subtle brain changes, or through the additive or interactive effects of both pathways.

Inhibitory control, therefore, is a crucial component of adaptive behavior that develops with the contributions of brain maturation and support from the environment. As will be discussed in the next section, it can be viewed as a component of executive functions, the cognitive processes dedicated to accomplishing future-oriented goals, as well as a mechanism for regulating arousal to function adaptively.

2.2 Inhibitory control as part of executive function and overall self-regulation

Nigg [11] developed a hierarchical model of self-regulation that attempted to reconcile several constructs in psychology that have been easily confused and often used interchangeably. Some of these constructs are executive function, effortful control, cognitive control, and emotional regulation. Nigg's model of self-regulation is designed to explain self-regulation in a domain-general manner. This would involve self-regulation over thought, action, and emotions, which fits well with our view of the importance of inhibitory control to all facets of adaptive behavior. The top-down processes of self-regulation are those that are deliberate and under the conscious control of the individual. These include basic executive functions such as inhibition, working memory, and flexibility, as well as effortful control needed to deal with conflicting demands. These top-down processes also include more complex cognitive control processes, such planning, reasoning, and other coping strategies, particularly those directed to regulating emotional arousal to allow cognitive control processes to be executed.

In Nigg's model, bottom-up processes include nervous system arousal that may reflect emotion, motivation, or stress responses. Typically, this arousal is adaptively controlled by the top-down regulatory processes, but arousal also may serve to energize self-regulation. As Blair and Raver [2] describe in the case of young children, bottom-up arousal often disrupts goal-directed behavior and, thus, requires top-down regulation. However, they point out that arousal can also facilitate adaptive behavior, as seen when a moderate level of stress improves performance [14] or when emotional tagging of memories improves encoding [15].

Therefore, inhibitory control fits within a complex web of executive function, effortful control and emotion regulation processes that are reciprocally connected to support overall self-regulation in service of adaptive behavior. Depending upon the individual's biological and learning history, and the contextual demands of the environment, inhibitory control and overall self-regulation will be challenged in a variety of ways. Individuals will vary widely in their self-regulatory abilities and these differences may be mediated by neurological differences and/or influenced by a range of life stress factors to which the individual has been exposed.

3. Brain systems underlying Self-regulation and inhibitory control

3.1 Relevant brain networks

The neurophysiological mediation of self-regulation represents the intersection of brain systems activated by bottom-up, "hot" sources of emotional and motivational arousal and the brain systems involved in "cool" cognitive control over that arousal for adaptive responses and decisions [16]. Emotional arousal is processed in the limbic system, particularly the amygdala, and strong motivational stimuli activates the reward system of the brain comprised of dopamine pathways and the limbic system structure, the nucleus accumbens [17]. The ventromedial portion of the prefrontal cortex serves to modulate the activity of the limbic system under conditions of strong arousal allowing the dorsolateral region of the prefrontal cortex to carry out its "cool" executive functions of planful, organized, and adaptive decision making [18]. Moreover, the right dorsolateral prefrontal cortex appears to be specifically involved in the inhibitory control aspect of executive function [19]. The smooth coordination of these various regions to appropriately react to arousing stimuli with a "fight or flight" response, as well as to mitigate such reactions when necessary to execute adaptive decision making, develops over the childhood and adolescent years [20]. Importantly, the prefrontal cortex shows the most protracted development from birth to adulthood of all cortical areas [21]. Thus, the plastic brain's vulnerability to biological and environmental insults related to life stress has critical implications for the development of inhibitory control and downstream difficulties with adaptive behavior.

3.2 Impacts of life stress on these brain regions

It is well-documented that chronic stress has deleterious effects on brain development and function, and many of the targets of stress are those networks involved in self-regulation, described above. Animal models, confirmed in human studies, have identified the dorsolateral prefrontal cortex, amygdala, and the ventromedial prefrontal cortex as consistent targets of the negative impacts of chronic stress on structure and function [22]. Stress-induced changes in the ventromedial prefrontal cortex have been specifically linked to cognitive control deficits in both animals and humans [23–25].

Prenatal and early postnatal development of the brain is the consequence of a complex unfolding of genetic and epigenetic mechanisms that can be derailed by adverse biological or environmental forces [26]. There is emerging evidence that poverty—with its many correlated stressors—is related to alterations in a variety of brain regions, including those related to self-regulation, the prefrontal cortex and amygdala [2]. Similarly, there is increasing evidence that childhood maltreatment, again correlated with poverty and other stressors, is related to alterations in the structure and function of brain networks involved in self-regulation. Research has identified the brain networks that differ in maltreated individuals as those that mediate emotional regulation, attention, inhibitory control, and social cognition, particularly in situations of threat or potential reward [27, 28].

Thus, the underlying brain mechanisms of self-regulation and inhibitory control are quite vulnerable to life adversity and stress, and this is likely to be observed in behavioral disruptions in high-risk individuals. In what follows, we discuss the evidence for impairments in inhibitory control, and related constructs of executive functions and self-regulation, that have been linked to four examples of life stress.

4. Life stress impacts on inhibitory control, executive function, and self-regulation

Life stress can include the mild, normative challenges that have been found to fine-tune the stress response system at the brain and behavioral levels to overcome obstacles and build resilience. Evolutionarily, our brains and bodies are equipped to deal with acute, short-lived stressors without serious negative consequences [29], but chronic, long-lasting, frequent, and/or extreme stress exposure results in what has been referred to as the toxic stress response [30]. Adverse childhood experiences, such as poverty, maltreatment, and parental conflict, are included in the category of toxic stress and have been found to disrupt inhibitory control, emotional regulation, and organized, reflective thinking [31, 32]. Individuals who contend with chronic life stress as adults may have also had exposure to toxic stress in their childhoods during the period of critical brain and behavioral development. As adults, these challenging conditions are likely to continue to impair the brain functions necessary for inhibitory control and overall self-regulation.

It is important to note that where there is risk, there is also substantial evidence of resilience in the face of adverse life circumstances, and this is observed both at the brain and behavioral levels [33]. Our own research has examined young adults with a childhood maltreatment history who manage to enroll in college [34] and homeless men who seek out services such as transitional housing [35]. These groups of adults are demonstrating resilience despite exposure to difficult and sometimes traumatic circumstances. While there is evidence of inhibitory control deficits in these groups, this capacity for resilience is likely to make these groups excellent candidates for interventions to strengthen inhibitory control and a range of related self-regulatory skills.

4.1 Poverty

According to 2017 data, almost 40 million people lived below the poverty line in the United States, and 12.8 million of this group were children [36]. Poverty is not a monolithic factor affecting psychological development; rather, poverty is correlated with numerous risk factors [37] that combine to create a cumulative risk to healthy development. Poverty-related risk factors that have a negative impact on the development of self-regulatory abilities in children include low maternal education, elevated maternal depression, exposure to domestic and neighborhood violence, lower housing quality, exposure to environmental pollutants, and poor access to needed services [38]. A gap in self-regulatory abilities is seen as early as preschool in low-income children [39], and growth in self-regulation is slower in impoverished children with a greater number of cumulative risks [40]. In a large, nationally-representative sample of children in Head Start, Son, Choi and Kwon [41] identified reciprocal associations between inhibitory control and math skills, and the researchers suggest that intervening to improve inhibitory control in low-income children will improve academic abilities, which in turn will improve self-regulation.

Poverty continues to negatively impact self-regulation beyond childhood. Lambert et al. [42] found that poverty was related to cognitive control deficits, while violence exposure was related to emotional dysregulation in a sample of adolescents. In a sample of more than 5000 adults 18–30 years of age, exposure to two decades or more of sustained poverty was related to poorer executive functions, which the researchers suggest have a negative impact on health-related behaviors and ultimately on longevity [43]. Poverty is a complex multifactorial construct that is clearly associated with many other risk factors, including those discussed below, which are themselves predictive of impairments in inhibitory control and related skills.

4.2 Childhood maltreatment

Based on data from the Centers for Disease Control and Prevention, approximately 1 in 7 U.S. children experience child abuse and/or neglect in the past year, and this statistic likely underestimates the scope of the problem [44]. Childhood maltreatment and other adverse experiences have been found to increase risks to physical health and overall adaptive functioning according to the well-known, large-scale Kaiser Foundation study [45]. Given the likely negative impacts on the developing brain and the altered learning environment of the child exposed to maltreatment, cognitive deficits and difficulties with self-regulation will potentially have life-long implications for adaptive behavior.

Evidence suggests impairments in a range of executive functions in childhood samples that have experienced maltreatment [46, 47]. Such deficits are also observed in adolescents and adults reporting a maltreatment history [48, 49]. Inhibitory control is frequently measured by the neurocognitive Go-No-Go task, which requires a response to a specific target and withholding a response (inhibition) to other targets. Adults self-reporting a history of abuse or neglect demonstrate difficulties with this task, particularly in the No-Go condition that demands inhibitory control [50, 51]. Such inhibitory control deficits may manifest as overall difficulties with self-regulation, placing adolescents and adults at risk for maladaptive behaviors and decision making [52].

4.3 Homelessness

As is the case for other adverse environmental conditions already discussed, homelessness is a serious societal problem; in January of 2015, it was estimated that there were 564,708 homeless people in the United States. Executive function impairments, among other cognitive deficits, are observed in youth who have experienced homelessness, foster care, and poverty according to a recent meta-analysis. For children experiencing homelessness, deficits in effortful and emotional control predict academic difficulties [53], and effortful control has also been found to be an individual resource contributing to overall adaptive functioning and resilience among these children [54]. Schmitt et al. [55] demonstrated that difficulties with inhibitory control mediated the relationship between housing insecurity and academic functioning of preschoolers. Thus, homelessness has a deleterious effect on the development of children particularly at a critical milestone of early academic adjustment and achievement, with potential negative impacts on later adaptation.

In adults, executive function skills, including inhibitory control, suffer substantially if a person experiences psychosocial stress [24], social exclusion [56, 57], interpersonal strain [58], or disrupted sleep [59], all of which are common among those experiencing homelessness. It is therefore not surprising that several studies have reported deficits in executive functions among homeless individuals including youth [60], adults [61], and older adults [62]. The experience of homelessness not only appears to put someone at risk for disrupted self-regulatory behaviors, such as executive function and inhibitory control, but these deficits also may result in maladaptive behavior that results in homelessness. Gabrielian et al. [63] compared the problem-solving skills homeless-experienced veterans in a US federal government study who retained ("stayers") or lost ("exiters") housing for at least 1 year. Both groups had poor cognition, but there was a trend toward greater problem-solving complexity in stayers as compared to exiters [64]. Similarly, in a study of the influence of cognition on community functioning among formerly homeless persons with mental illness, better executive functions predicted improved self-care and less turbulent behavior [65].

In the United States, the prevalent problem of homelessness among military veterans merits particular attention. Veterans are at particularly high risk of homelessness for several reasons including relatively disadvantaged socioeconomic status and increased risk of mental disorders, both of which are associated with impairments in executive functions (as discussed in Sections 4.1 and 4.4, respectively) [66, 67].

As will be discussed in Section 6, there is a need to carefully consider the role of executive functions in homeless veterans with and without mental illness, both as a potential cause and consequence of these problems, and to develop interventions tailored to the needs of this vulnerable population.

4.4 Mental illness

There is evidence on both brain and behavioral levels that cognitive and emotional regulation deficits may be transdiagnostic symptoms; that is, these difficulties are found across a range of mental illness diagnosis in children and adults. Maladaptive decision-making behavior is observed in youth with anxiety, depression, conduct disorder, and ADHD, though the particular manifestations of these deficits may vary [68]. A meta-analysis by Wright et al. [69] identified small-to-moderate deficits in inhibitory control on tasks such as the Go-No-Go across 11 different mental illness diagnoses in adults. In adolescents with a history of depression, specific deficits in inhibitory control were still observed even after remission of their depression, while other executive functions and cognitive abilities had improved.

Adults with serious mental illness (schizophrenia, schizoaffective disorder, bipolar disorder, major depressive disorder, and posttraumatic stress disorder) frequently exhibit impairments in executive function and cognitive control [70, 71]. Notably, executive functions have been shown to be the most important cognitive domain for a variety of adaptive outcomes for individuals with serious mental illness, including occupational functioning and independent living [72]. Similarly, difficulties with executive functions and overall self-regulation predict maladaptive outcomes in these mentally ill adults, such as treatment nonadherence and violent behavior [72], poor treatment response [73], and overall psychosocial function [74].

In summary, severe life stresses such as poverty, childhood maltreatment, homelessness, and mental illness have adverse effects on the self-regulatory processes such as executive function and inhibitory control. In many cases such stresses co-occur, with cumulative negative effects. Inhibitory control is critical to adaptive functioning across a wide range of domains: academic, employment, interpersonal, and physical and mental health. Stressful life circumstances can create a cascade effect on self-regulatory capacities that may lead to maladaptive behavioral consequences such as risky or antisocial behavior. In turn, maladaptive behaviors place the individual in environments that continue to limit the development of these important skills. For example, an adolescent who engages in delinquent behaviors with peers will not have the role models or the learning experiences to shape appropriate inhibitory control or executive functions in the future. As will be described later in the chapter, US military veterans frequently experience a combination of these stresses when they return home (e.g., homelessness and mental illness) and are at great risk for difficulties with self-regulation. Thus, due to the biological and environmental risk factors that may contribute to deficits in these critical skills in a substantial minority of the population, interventions that can ameliorate these difficulties should hold promise for substantial benefits for both the individual and society.

5. Interventions for inhibitory control and executive function

5.1 Growing interest in prevention intervention

Scientists are using increasingly advanced techniques to study the brain, behavior, and interventions for improving health [75–77]. Findings include

Nobel-prize-winning research that demonstrates how the brain forms synapses when it learns something new [78], the identification of executive functions that are learned through practice [79–81], and research indicating the brain continues to produce neurons well into old age [82].

These and other studies support and complement research showing that thinking skills are learned behaviors and that when they are not developed, are only partially learned, or are compromised by adversity and stress, they negatively impact the physical and mental health of individuals, families, and communities [26, 75, 77, 83]. We know that most mental health disorders and problems are largely preventable. This knowledge underlies requests from health providers, educators, and concerned citizens for access to research and prevention programs [76, 84]. In the last two decades, a greater number of scientific papers has been published on prevention programs [85], biological and social behavior interventions [76], and self-control and intertemporal choice in economics [86]. They reflect the diverse and valuable advances in research on a wide range of approaches that address prevention to promote healthy life choices.

5.2 BrainWise program

The BrainWise program is a prevention curriculum that uses a multidisciplinary approach to teach 10 thinking skills that include inhibitory control and other executive functions [35]. The program focuses on neurocognitive development and integrates findings from social science, education, and neuroscience. It integrates the roles that the prefrontal cortex and limbic system play in decision making, explains them simply, and provides a template for teaching thinking skills.

Program participants are students and clients of diverse ages, backgrounds, and abilities. The program uses nonscientific terms to explain basic brain processes and provides scripted lessons, making the material easy to understand and remember by children, youth, and adults, including individuals with disabilities and mental health challenges [87, 88]. BrainWise instructors can adapt scientific terms to fit their students' and clients' level of understanding whether the individuals are learning disabled or high performers.

The curriculum uses activities that combine kinesthetic, sensory-motor, visual, auditory, cognitive, and socioemotional techniques instructors can adapt and customize as needed. Its approach includes teaching basic brain concepts using activities that engage participants of all ages, helping them understand why learning and practicing enables them to stop and think before they act. The program can be adapted to address a wide range of teaching situations and can be taught in classes, small groups, and one-on-one. This flexibility appeals to instructors and helps ensure they will teach and reinforce the lessons with fidelity [89, 90]. Instructors learn how to integrate the lessons into daily activities, providing opportunities to use examples that are specific to problems faced by their clients and students.

Reinforcement is key to retention [76, 91–94]. Instructors have access to several BrainWise teaching aids and create their own. These include problem-solving worksheets, checklists, reinforcement games, and support activities that sometimes call for older students to teach and reinforce lessons with younger students. Depending on the site and instructor, text messages, apps, telephone, emails, and other devices are additional reinforcement strategies. For example, instructors may randomly send customized text messages to remind a participant to "Exit Your Emotions Elevator" or "Use Your Wizard Brain!". Course instructors also have access to a "members-only" BrainWise network where they share teaching strategies and techniques and receive a monthly online newsletter containing research updates, teaching tips, and instructors' stories.

DOI: http://dx.doi.org/10.5772/intechopen.88642

BrainWise is taught in schools, clinics, faith-based organizations, agencies, worksites, homeless shelters, hospitals, and households throughout the United States and in Canada, China, India, and 17 other countries [95]. U.S. Indian Health Services (IHS) has recognized BrainWise as a program that benefits Native Americans and Alaska natives, and the University of Tennessee Extension has trained its agents to teach BrainWise throughout the state [96]. The advocacy of program users underlies this growth, and a future direction for application of BrainWise will be to incarcerated youth and adults.

5.3 The 10 Wise Ways

BrainWise starts with four tenets: (1) everyone has problems; (2) people who have fewer problems use thinking skills; (3) the brain can help prevent problems; and (4) the 10 Wise Ways teach thinking skills. This section presents the lessons and research supporting each one (**Figure 1**).

5.3.1 Wise Way 1: use your Wizard Brain over your Lizard Brain

This statement lays the foundation for the nine lessons that follow. Participants learn how the body's five senses act as sentinels and send signals to the brain's thalamus, which is also called the relay center because it collects sensory information and sends it to the limbic system to be processed.

The limbic system is located beneath the relay center and contains the amygdala (where fear and any intense emotion are triggered) and the hypothalamus (which sets off the fight or flight reaction; [97]). These survival responses are also found in reptiles, leading us to call this section the Lizard Brain. Instructors use this information to discuss the history and importance of survival instincts and how the amygdala (emotion center) and hypothalamus (fight or flight reaction) contribute to impulsive reactions, such as maladaptive road rage [98].

Participants receive worksheets with age-appropriate pictures of brains and label the parts as they learn about them. They see the Lizard Brain's proximity to the brain stem. They learn that the part of the brain behind the forehead contains the thinking area known as the prefrontal cortex. For simplicity, we call it the Wizard Brain and point out that all of us are born with only rudimentary connections from the relay center to the Wizard Brain. These connections develop as we learn, Sapolsky [76] discusses the neurobiological stages involved in top-down, Wizard Brain decision-making.

Wise Way #1 *Wizard Brain Over Your Lizard Brain*	**Wise Way #2** *Build a Constellation of Support*	**Wise Way #3** *Red Flag Warnings*	**Wise Way #4** *Exit the Emotions Elevator*	**Wise Way #5** *Fact vs Opinion*
Wise Way #6 *Ask Questions and Gather Information*	**Wise Way #7** *Identify Choices (IDC)*	**Wise Way #8** *Consider Consequences Now and Later*	**Wise Way #9** *Set Goals and Plans for Action*	**Wise Way #10** *Communicate Effectively*

Figure 1.
The 10 Wise Ways.

This sets the stage for presenting a powerful piece of information. The skills participants learn in BrainWise help them build connections to their Wizard Brain so that when signals are sent to the relay center, they are diverted away from the Lizard Brain and to the Wizard Brain. This simplified explanation is easy for almost anyone to understand [35]. Each time participants learns a wise way, they draw a line from the relay center/Lizard Brain to the Wizard Brain. This process helps participants of all ages and abilities form a clear picture of how different parts of the brain respond to a stimulus.

Wise Way 1 lays the foundation for the remaining skills by helping participants learn how the brain is involved in behaviors and what they can do to prevent and manage problems. As discussed in the previous section, the hierarchical model of self-regulation developed by Nigg [11] describes these processes as "top-down" and "bottom-up." The top-down processes are Wizard Brain responses that include executive functions and the complex planning, reasoning, and other coping strategies taught throughout the remaining Wise Ways. The bottom-up processes are all Lizard Brain reactions to events that arouse strong emotions. These will be addressed in Wise Ways 2–10.

The lesson ends with participants drawing a line on the brain worksheet to show that Wise Way 1 helps them make a connection. Sapolsky [76] presents this process in a discussion about how the ventromedial prefrontal cortex forms connections with the limbic system, and the biological processes underlying such neuroplasticity are presented by Kandel [78].

5.3.2 Wise Way 2: build a Constellation of Support

Research supports the importance of human connection [99–102] and identifies how support systems can be lifelines out of loneliness, helplessness, sadness, and other feelings of being isolated. Wise Way 2 helps people learn how to create and use an effective support network by teaching about resources for different types of support, as well as how to find and access dependable support sources.

Participants learn to identify a wider range of sources they can go to for help, a process that increases their awareness of the benefits of sources they previously may not have considered. This includes learning that valued help takes many forms—human, animal, spiritual, and inanimate—and that we all need to identify and access different types of support for our various problems [103, 104].

The Constellation of Support shows that we connect with the "stars" in our constellation in three ways: (1) Broken Line (not helpful), (2) Single Line (not unhelpful, but not helpful either), or (3) Double Lines (helpful). This activity creates awareness that broken lines may include unthinking friends and family, members with their own set of problems who do not realize that alternative help is available or how to access it. The course instructor is always a double line for the client or student and is a resource for other support sources. This lesson and visual teaching activities are valuable tools that help participants assess the degree of help a support resource provides.

The science of social support is complex and involves many biological pathways, including neuropeptides, genes, and hormones [76, 105]. These studies are consistent with the advantages of utilizing resources and support, a concept that is taught as a key connection to the Wizard Brain. Participants learn that the Constellation of Support is complicated, and resources can be deceptive, potentially causing problems instead of preventing them if one is not careful. The lesson makes individuals aware that help is always available and the skills they are learning will help them access the most useful sources.

5.3.3 Wise Way 3: Red Flag Warnings

Teaching about Red Flag Warnings builds on what participants learned about the Lizard Brain's bottom-up arousal. The body's five senses continuously receive sensory cues, and this lesson creates awareness of signals that warn "something is going to happen." Individuals learn about their unique sensations warning of problems and the importance of recognizing two types: External Red Flags and Internal Red Flags.

External Red Flags are audio signals, such as a siren, or visual cues, such as gang colors or empty beer cans on the front porch. Participants learn to identify how they react to red flags, especially in problem situations. This recognition creates an awareness of maladaptive behaviors. For example, one client realized that he would turn his head and spit immediately before he lost his temper. When he recognized this as an external warning signal, he was able to control his behavior.

Internal Red Flags are what a person feels inside, a key component of emotion regulation. Participants may say, "I feel mad," or name emotions such as frustration, sadness, loneliness, and unhappiness. Instructors ask them to describe what they feel inside, probing to identify physical sensations such as tight muscles, hot flashes, and upset stomach. Helping them become aware of internal red flags is as important for 5-year-olds as it is for older youth and adults. Instructors and parents find that students with ADHD and autism can learn to identify internal sensations they may feel before an emotional or physical incident.

The Red Flag Warnings content includes teaching aids and activities that promote reinforcement. Participants, including adults, make personalized red flags and list their Internal Red Flags on one side and External Red Flags on the other. Young children complete Red Flag Buddy worksheets, marking areas where they feel red flags. This awareness helps prepare them for times when sensory information streams toward their brains and rapidly, powerfully, and automatically triggers behaviors [85].

After they learn the lesson, they draw a line on the brain worksheet showing that they are building another connection to their Wizard Brain. This seemingly simple process puts into practice the neuroscience behind emotions and impulse [76] and gives instructors a segue to the next lesson on emotions and how to control them.

5.3.4 Wise Way 4: exit the Emotions Elevator

The Constellation of Support and Red Flag Warnings lessons prepare participants to learn about their emotions and techniques to control them using their Wizard Brain. The first part of the lesson explains emotions by using the metaphor of an elevator, but instructors can use metaphors that may be more familiar to their students; e.g., instructors in rural China and India use fires and volcanoes, so participants create individualized Emotions Elevators.

In the context of teaching Wise Way 4, participants learn the following: (1) Emotions are cumulative and have a range of intensity [22]. BrainWise teaches that the first floor is low emotion and the higher floors are out of control. (2) Multiple emotions are experienced simultaneously, e.g., one can be enraged but also feel admiration for a worthy adversary. Additionally, participants learn that emotions can be on different floors of the Elevator—one can be scared, but also extremely curious and excited; extreme emotions, from one to many, hijack Wizard Brain thinking and replace it with Lizard Brain impulse. (3) Any emotion that is high on the elevator triggers Lizard Brain reactions, from being "crazy in love" to taking a selfie in a dangerous location [76].

They also learn that it is difficult to impossible to stop emotions when they hit the high floors of the Emotions Elevator. Lizard Brain reactions are swift, from uttering hateful words to acting in anger. Participants learn to distinguish between helpful emotions and toxic emotions and are taught that skills help them control their emotions to decrease stress and promote healthy behaviors [24, 31].

The second part of the lesson teaches them how to stay off their Emotions Elevators or how to stay on the lower floors, so they can access the Wizard Brain. These techniques include strategies that help control emotions such as control self-talk, stop talking, leave the situation, redirect your emotions, and control relaxation. Instructors are encouraged to add any number of interventions that will help their clients and students regulate inhibition and improve self-control [85, 106, 107]. BrainWise helps participants recognize that many strategies are available and use the Wizard Brain to find what works best for them.

Skills to exit the Emotions Elevator are taught as behaviors used to promote Wizard Brain thinking and help participants build neural pathways to reroute Lizard Brain impulses. This process builds on Wise Ways 1–3 and lays a foundation for subsequent lessons.

5.3.5 Wise Way 5: Fact vs. Opinion

Fake news has existed for a long time. Parkinson [108] describes the propaganda, cooked-up stories, and hoaxes deliberately planted by Benjamin Franklin, John Adams, Nathaniel Hawthorne, and other Revolutionary leaders to instill fear in colonists against the British, Indians, and African Americans. Instructors have no shortage of examples of falsehoods and half-truths from past and present history as well as daily events in the participants' lives.

Research conducted by the Stanford History Education Group (SHEG) with 7804 middle school, high school and college students in 12 states found that students have a "dismaying" inability to tell fake news from real news [109]. SHEG is working with educators to create materials that help young people navigate the fake news they encounter online. These are the kinds of resources BrainWise instructors use to teach and reinforce Fact vs. Opinion.

These lessons promote awareness of the role emotions play in fostering Lizard Brain actions and spark discussion on how using Wise Ways 1–4 puts questionable information into perspective. At the end of the lesson, participants draw a line on the brain worksheet to show they have learned another skill to help them use their Wizard Brain to prevent and solve problems. Instructors encourage them to reinforce the lesson by applying the skill to relationships, work, and current events.

5.3.6 Wise Way 6: ask questions and gather information

Asking the right questions helps people separate facts from opinions. Participants recognize that learning to ask good questions involves using their Wizard Brain, being off (or low on) their Emotions Elevators and accessing reliable sources in their Constellation of Support. Participants may have little or no experience stopping to think about the information they need. The lesson is a primer on obtaining facts and helps individuals practice gathering them effectively. This skill strengthens the neural networks that help the Wizard Brain to regulate the emotional arousal of the Lizard Brain transition [76]. At the conclusion of the lesson, participants add another line to their brain worksheet, creating a visual reminder that the skills they are learning will help divert Lizard Brain impulses.

5.3.7 Wise Way 7: Identify choices (IDC)

Individuals dependent on their Lizard Brain often feel victimized. They are clueless about other choices because the limbic system's rapid-fire reactions drive their behavior and blind them to other choices they could make. The high intensity of their anger, sadness, despair, hopelessness, or other emotions they experience overcomes them, making it impossible to consider other choices [22]. Even if they want to make good choices, they fail to follow through [110].

Exploring all of one's choices is a new concept for participants who rely mainly on their Lizard Brains. To bolster awareness of identifying and making choices, instructors ask participants to generate as many choices as they can, positive and negative, for problem situations. They are reminded to include "not making a choice." This activity helps change myopic perceptions that cause problems. Ericson and Laibson [107] discuss how myopic behavior creates "cognitive noise" that causes perceptual limitations. Wise Way 7 helps participants expand their thinking about choices and prepares them for the next skill—considering the consequences of making a choice.

5.3.8 Wise Way 8: consider consequences

For many participants, considering consequences is a missing step. Learning the skill and using it can be an "Aha!" moment for them. People who have never learned consequential thinking fall back on Lizard Brain impulses. Being aware not only that they have choices, but that they can determine the best choice by considering the consequences now and later (CNL) and the consequences affecting others (CAO) gives them options they never knew they had.

Thinking about the outcomes of choices is complicated [2, 76, 107]. This lesson teaches consequential thinking in the context of the seven preceding skills. It provides a framework that helps individuals put the lessons together as part of the Wizard Brain thinking that usurps harmful Lizard Brain reactions. Considering the impact of choices involves future thinking (i.e., executive functions) and inhibitory control, instructors may use this introduction to expand the lesson to discussions of mental health, diets, the environment, relationships, education, and finances.

One teenager referred to CNL as the "thinking skill that saved my life." She said she was considering committing suicide and did not follow through because she thought about the consequences her death would have on her mother. She wrote her teacher a testimonial about the incident. Another student at her school had recently committed suicide, and we are grateful she did not repeat the act. Her positive choice is supported by research showing that people who are suicidal or self-injure have decreased neurocognitive functions and an absence of inhibitory control [111].

Lizard Brain dominance eliminates consequential thinking as emotions hijack thinking. Sadly, we know that even strong Wizard Brain connections are not a guarantee against harmful behaviors, but they are helpful for prevention and intervention. When participants draw lines on their brain worksheets indicating they have learned another connection, they know that practice strengthens the connections. They also begin to recognize positive results they attribute to using their Wizard Brain.

5.3.9 Wise Way 9: set goals and plans for action

Translating goals to behaviors requires using multiple Wise Ways. People who have never been taught how to apply goal setting to achieve success—graduating, losing weight, making friends, getting sober—often rely on Lizard Brain reactions that sabotage their good intentions and lead to failure. Their high Emotions Elevator excitement may not be directed in an adaptive manner to get sober, lose weight, exercise, or achieve whatever goal they set, and instead it fuels a greater desire to drink, eat, and give up.

Industries have been built around goal setting and ways to motivate people to change and sustain behaviors. Even people who have thinking skills are stymied by powerful emotions that destroy goals. This lesson creates awareness of the delicate balance between the Wizard Brain and Lizard Brain. Our brains can be tricky, and it helps when people understand how to obtain resources, why Lizard Brain responses can dominate, and what boosts Wizard Brain thinking. Participants learn that people who achieve their goals know how to manage the bottom-up Lizard Brain urges with top-down Wizard Brain skills. These lessons, activities, and problem-solving worksheets are additional tools that help participants use their brains to make good choices.

5.3.10 Wise Way 10: communicate effectively

This skill is taught at the end of the course because its successful implementation requires knowledge and use of the preceding nine Wise Ways. It is divided into three sections: verbal communication, nonverbal communication, and assertive communication.

The teaching activities include participant role plays that demonstrate using "I" messages, sending double messages, taking other people's point of view, and discussing the simultaneous use of communication with other Wise Ways. Participants learn to differentiate between assertive communication behaviors and passive, aggressive, and passive-aggressive behaviors. The lesson includes discussions about replacing Lizard Brain reactions with Wizard Brain behaviors, using support resources, recognizing red flag warnings, understanding the role emotions play, separating fact from opinion, asking questions, identifying choices, and setting goals.

Participants draw the tenth line on their brain worksheet to show that they have learned how to build another brain connection. They know that if they do not practice and use the skills, the links to the Wizard Brain weaken and disappear and are quickly replaced by Lizard Brain reactions.

The BrainWise curriculum was developed for nonscientists—the children, youth, and adults who take the course to learn skills that will help them make healthy decisions. It presents information in an easily understood format, so that it will be practiced until the skills and behaviors are automatic and retained [112]. Retention indicates mastery of the 10 Wise Ways. Program graduates are aware of the difference between Lizard Brain and Wizard Brain behaviors and have skills that make it easier to choose healthy behaviors.

5.4 BrainWise efficacy with populations exposed to childhood maltreatment and poverty—research with schools and families

Consistent, positive results have been reported on evaluations conducted across a variety of populations by different researchers. Participants in these studies include children living below the poverty line who have experienced multiple Adverse Childhood Experiences (ACEs), including maltreatment. A primary context for studying the effectiveness of BrainWise has been in schools identified as "at-risk." One study compared a group of inner-city middle school students who were taught BrainWise with a matched control group. The results found that students who took BrainWise demonstrated significant changes in decreasing physical aggression, reducing negative feelings, and increasing peer acceptance. They also showed improvements on a belief scale and moral order scale. The control group showed no changes. A student described the program by stating, "It doesn't change the person. It changes how the person thinks" [113]. In another study described by Barry and Welsh [95], students given the BrainWise curriculum in schools in a large metropolitan district were administered executive function tasks, Tower of London and Stroop, in a pre-post design. The findings indicated students who learned BrainWise showed improvements on the measures, and knowledge of the 10 Wise Ways also was related to self-reported executive function skills [113]. Pre- and post-data also were collected on 539 K–5 students who took BrainWise. Teachers rated the children on goal-oriented behavior, decision-making, emotional regulation, self-management, self-awareness, and relationship skills. Significant improvements were noted on all measures [114].

The efficacy of the BrainWise curriculum also has been demonstrated in public health contexts. Research was conducted on BrainWise by public health nurses working with at-risk families at a state agency. All the families had more than one child and presented risk behaviors and health problems: some had histories of child abuse, 75% were single parents with less than 12 years of education, and 61% were unemployed. The nurses visited the families a minimum of four times and measured outcomes using a Life Skills Progression checklist. Following each visit, the nurse used the checklist to measure parental behaviors. Data collected on 112 families found improvement on all 39 life-skill variables and significant improvement on 24 variables [115].

5.5 BrainWise efficacy with homeless men

There is a small, emerging literature on the effect of homelessness on neuropsychological impairment, including the evidence discussed in Section 4.3, but studies with comparison groups are rare [116]. We conducted a study of the BrainWise program delivered to homeless men at a transitional housing facility [35]. The homeless organization serving the men in our study presented a rare opportunity to conduct research with a comparison group. The men in both groups had progressed from the intake phase to transitional housing, indicating high motivation to change the behaviors that contributed to their homelessness.

The treatment group (N = 210) was taught BrainWise in Phase 1 of the treatment that included services such as counseling and case management, along with classes in life skills, career training, education, and spiritual development. The control group (N = 66) received all the services and classes with the exception of BrainWise. A staff counselor taught BrainWise and customized the examples using problems and situations typical of those the men faced. She consolidated the lessons and taught them during the first week of the men's placement. She reinforced the concepts outside the classroom during her daily interactions with the men. Other staff and volunteers received training in BrainWise and reinforced the lessons during their interactions with the men.

The men completed pretests and posttests on validated instruments that included eight scales measuring executive functions (Behavior Rating Scale for Executive Function, or BRIEF), one scale measuring coping self-efficacy (Coping Self-Efficacy Scale, or CSES), a self-report on problem solving skills (Wasik Problem Solving Rating Scale, or WPSRS), and a scale that measured participants' knowledge of the thinking and emotional skills taught in BrainWise (BrainWise Knowledge Survey, or BKS). These instruments were found to be reliable for a sample unaccustomed to taking such measures. They were administered the posttest 4 months after learning the 10 Wise Ways.

The results demonstrated that the men in the treatment group improved on a much wider range of executive functions (including inhibitory control), coping self-efficacy, and BrainWise knowledge than the men in the comparison group. This provided evidence that BrainWise positively influences critical skills for adaptive functioning and resilience. These improved skills and knowledge will likely help them better face the many daily challenges, such as maintaining healthy relationships, holding jobs, and becoming productive members of society [35].

6. Vulnerable veteran populations and the BrainWise intervention

6.1 Veteran homelessness and serious mental illness

The promising results of the preceding study have given rise to an effort to study the implementation of BrainWise within the U.S. Department of Veterans Affairs (VA). Homelessness among veterans is a sizeable and urgent problem and addressing it is a high priority for VA. According to the 2018 Annual Homeless Assessment Report (AHAR) to Congress, nearly 38,000 Veterans in the U.S. were experiencing homelessness on a single night, of whom roughly 14,500 were completely unsheltered [115]. The cornerstone of the VA's efforts to reduce veteran homelessness is the Housing and Urban Development–Veterans Affairs Supported Housing (HUD-VASH) program, which provides housing subsidies and case management services to eligible veterans. HUD-VASH has been instrumental in reducing the nation's homeless veteran population, which dropped by 52% from 2009 to 2018 [117]. However, many veterans in the program fail to obtain housing, and many who do subsequently return to homelessness [118]. Clearly, despite access to similar resources, many veterans are not succeeding. While the reasons for this are complex, individual characteristics account for some of these disparate outcomes. In particular, serious mental illnesses such as schizophrenia and bipolar disorder [119, 120] and substance use disorders [121] are major risk factors for homelessness among veterans.

6.2 Combat-related risk factors for executive dysfunction

Given disproportionate rates of mental illness among Veterans, the impairments in executive functions related to a variety of psychiatric conditions discussed in Section 4.4 are especially relevant to this population [67]. In addition, veterans are at unique risk for combat-related posttraumatic stress disorder (PTSD) and traumatic brain injury (TBI). PTSD and TBI, which frequently co-occur, are considered signature conditions of the wars in Iraq and Afghanistan due to their high prevalence among this cohort [122]. PTSD is associated with impaired executive function irrespective of current symptom severity [123]. Similarly, because the frontal lobes are particularly susceptible to traumatic injury, deficits in executive function are common sequelae of TBI, even in mild cases [124]. Rabinowitz and Levin highlight the negative impact of moderate to severe TBI on judgment and everyday decision making, suggesting a possible role for the BrainWise program given its emphasis on and approach to decision making skills [125]. Specifically, TBI can disrupt the process of associating visceral emotional responses with positive and negative outcomes. TBI impacts several aspects of decision making, including impulsivity, risk adjustment, and rational choice, owing to abnormalities in the anatomic regions responsible for each of these functions [126]. Although untested in this regard, the BrainWise program's emphasis on strengthening systems of emotional control and reinforcing neural pathways involved in adaptive decision making may be well suited as a rehabilitative strategy for persons with TBI.

6.3 Conceptual model of executive functions and veteran homelessness

As previously discussed in Sections 4.1–4.4, homelessness itself, predisposing factors for homelessness such as poverty and childhood maltreatment, factors resulting from homelessness such as stress and social exclusion, psychiatric illness in general, and veteran-specific conditions such as combat PTSD and TBI are all associated with impairments in executive functions. Many individuals are burdened by several of these factors. In turn, there is evidence that executive functions mediate several processes may which impact a person's ability to obtain housing and remain housed, such as risk-taking behaviors, conduct problems (e.g., violent behavior), and aspects of self-care. Taken together, a conceptual model begins to emerge by which we can represent some of the relationships between executive function, factors that impact it, and its effect on housing outcomes (**Figure 2**).

The symbols indicate positive (+) and negative (−) associations. As shown in the model, executive functions appear to have both direct and indirect effects on housing stability. For example, poor planning can lead directly to loss of housing (e.g., via failure to pay rent), and poor inhibitory control can lead to behaviors such as substance use and conduct problems which then lead to housing loss. Of note, a number of possible points of intervention within the model are addressed by existing VA services—treatment of mental illness, TBI, and substance use, provision of housing services, and case management to address psychosocial needs—but a focus on executive functions is not among these. The possibility of intervening to improve executive functions presents an opportunity to augment existing VA services with the aim of improving housing outcomes for homeless veterans. BrainWise was selected for this purpose because it is the only program known to have evidence for improving executive functions in homeless individuals.

6.4 Adaptation of BrainWise for homeless veterans with serious mental illness

The chapter authors, working with other investigators at VA, have developed a proposal to adapt the BrainWise curriculum for use with homeless and recently homeless veterans diagnosed with serious mental illness, using input from VA staff and veterans themselves. The initial pilot study would be carried out at the Greater Los Angeles VA Medical Center, in an integrated care clinic for homeless veterans called a Homeless Patient-Aligned Care Team (HPACT). HPACT services include primary care, mental health and substance use treatment, and case management, with care tailored to the unique needs of homeless veterans. The HPACT model has resulted in a number of positive outcomes [121, 127] and presents an opportune

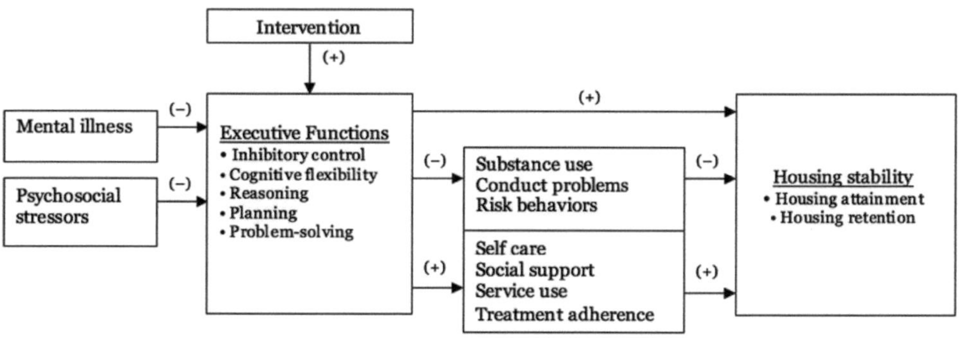

Figure 2.
Conceptual model of life stress, executive functions and housing stability.

venue for implementation of innovations that fill service gaps. The design and procedures of this proposed pilot study are described, below.

During an initial adaptation phase, the research team interview key stakeholders consisting of clinicians and administrators in the HPACT clinic and HUD-VASH program, as well as homeless veterans from an established Veteran Engagement Group. The BrainWise program and materials are described and shown to the stakeholders, who are then asked to provide input regarding aspects of the curriculum that appear most and least relevant, barriers or problems they anticipate in delivering the intervention, situations homeless veterans face which could be used as teaching examples, and other suggestions or thoughts they may have. The interviews are recorded, transcribed, and analyzed using qualitative research methods in order to identify salient themes and extract information to be used to guide the initial adaptation of the BrainWise materials.

The adapted curriculum is taught in a series of weekly sessions to two groups of approximately 8–12 HPACT patients diagnosed with schizophrenia or other forms of psychosis, with or without a substance use disorder. Immediately following each intervention session, participants provide feedback on the session, and this information is recorded, analyzed, used to conduct further modifications of the curriculum based on input from participants. At the same time, the research team monitors the fidelity of the adapted curriculum to assure that core BrainWise elements are retained.

In addition to the development of content and format tailored to this population, the key outcomes of interest for this pilot study are the feasibility and acceptability of the intervention for the population of homeless veterans with psychotic disorders. We would also gather preliminary data on the effects of the intervention on executive functions, BrainWise content knowledge, substance use, and housing trajectory, by assessing these variables prior to and immediately following the intervention course. Although such results are not intended to be conclusive due to the lack of a control group and the small number of participants planned for the initial study, conducting these assessments would provide valuable information about the feasibility of the data collection methods in this population. It would also yield descriptive statistics that would assist in planning a larger controlled trial of the adapted BrainWise curriculum. Our hope is that this work may form the foundation for the wide-scale incorporation of BrainWise programming into homeless services throughout VA, and more importantly that the tools gained from the program can help these vulnerable veterans emerge from homelessness and more successfully navigate their everyday lives.

7. Conclusions

Researchers continue to explore the diverse manifestations of inhibitory control across development, as well as its importance to the adaptive domains of executive functions and self-regulation. The brain systems critical to the normal development of these skills are guided by genetic and epigenetic phenomenon, as well as supported by an environment that provides learning opportunities and age-appropriate challenges. However, it is also clear that the brain systems underlying inhibitory control are vulnerable to a variety of stressors, which can result is differences in developmental trajectories and functioning. Research also confirms that such life stressors as poverty, childhood maltreatment, homelessness, and mental illness, are associated with impaired functioning in inhibitory control, executive functions, and overall self-regulation.

In this chapter, we introduced the BrainWise program as a universal curriculum that translates basic biological science to prevention skills taught by educators and health providers. We discussed how its approach optimizes findings on effective interventions, simplifies their delivery, and integrates them with brain science. The section described the 10 skills instructors teach to students and clients and the scientific support for each one, and presented research that had been conducted with children, adolescents, and adults.

We gave examples of how the program has been successfully used with elementary, middle, and high school students as well as families on welfare and homeless-experienced men, shared research on the program's outcomes, and provided access to additional resources. The information provided a template showing how science can be scaled to develop lessons that teach thinking skills to diverse populations and reach individuals who will benefit from learning executive functions, including inhibitory control and emotional regulation.

Finally, we suggest an application of the BrainWise curriculum to a very vulnerable population of veterans with serious mental illness, and potential TBI, who have experienced homelessness. The simplicity and accessibility of this intervention to a wide range of circumstances, as well as it's focus on some key executive function impairments in this population make this a promising direction for inquiry. At-risk and high-risk populations of individuals incur personal and societal costs of poor decision making and impulsive behaviors which may be ameliorated by appropriate, targeted, and flexible neurocognitive interventions.

Author details

Marilyn Welsh[1]*, Patricia Gorman Barry[2] and Jared M. Greenberg[3,4]

1 School of Psychological Sciences, University of Northern Colorado, Greeley, CO, USA

2 BrainWise, Denver, CO, USA

3 Jane and Terry Semel Institute for Neuroscience and Human Behavior at UCLA, Department of Psychiatry and Biobehavioral Sciences, David Geffen School of Medicine, University of California, Los Angeles, Los Angeles, CA, USA

4 VA Health Services Research and Development Center for the Study of Healthcare Innovation, Implementation, and Policy, VA Greater Los Angeles Healthcare System, Los Angeles, CA, USA

*Address all correspondence to: marilyn.welsh@unco.edu

References

[1] Sameroff A. A unified theory of development: A dialectic integration of nature and nurture. Child Development. 2010;**81**(1):6-22. DOI: 10.1111/j.1467-8624.2009.01378.x

[2] Blair C, Raver CC. Poverty, stress, and brain development: New directions for prevention and intervention. Academic Pediatrics. 2016;**16**(3):S30-S36. DOI: 10.1016/j.acap.2016.01.010

[3] Gilmore C, Attridge N, Clayton S, et al. Individual differences in inhibitory control, not non-verbal number acuity, correlate with mathematics achievement. PLoS One. 2013;**8**(6). DOI: 10.1371/journal.pone.0067374

[4] Houde' O, Borst GG. Measuring inhibitory control in children and adults: Brain imaging and mental chronometry. Frontiers in Psychology. 2014;**5**:1-7. DOI: 10.3389/fpsyg.2014.00616

[5] Shulman EP, Smith AR, Silva K, et al. The dual systems model: Review, reappraisal, and reaffirmation. Developmental Cognitive Neuroscience. 2016;**17**:103-117. DOI: 10.1016/j.dcn.2015.12.010

[6] Geurts HM, Van Den Bergh SFWM, Ruzzano L. Prepotent response inhibition and interference control in autism spectrum disorders: Two meta-analyses. Autism Research. 2014;**7**(4):407-420. DOI: 10.1002/aur.1369

[7] Padmanabhan A, Garver K, O'Hearn K, et al. Developmental changes in brain function underlying inhibitory control in autism spectrum disorders. Autism Research. 2014;**8**(2):123-135. DOI: 10.1002/aur.1398

[8] Fan L-Y, Gau SS-F, Chou T-L. Neural correlates of inhibitory control and visual processing in youths with attention deficit hyperactivity disorder: A counting Stroop functional MRI study. Psychological Medicine. 2014;**44**(12):2661-2671. DOI: 10.1017/s0033291714000038

[9] Geurts HM, Oord SVD, Crone EA. Hot and cool aspects of cognitive control in children with ADHD: Decision-making and inhibition. Journal of Abnormal Child Psychology. 2006;**34**(6):811-822. DOI: 10.1007/s10802-006-9059-2

[10] Woltering S, Lishak V, Hodgson N, Granic I, Zelazo PD. Executive function in children with externalizing and comorbid internalizing behavior problems. Journal of Child Psychology and Psychiatry. 2015;**57**(1):30-38. DOI: 10.1111/jcpp.12428

[11] Nigg JT. Annual research review: On the relations among self-regulation, self-control, executive functioning, effortful control, cognitive control, impulsivity, risk-taking, and inhibition for developmental psychopathology. Journal of Child Psychology and Psychiatry. 2016;**58**(4):361-383. DOI: 10.1111/jcpp.12675

[12] Mischel W, Shoda Y, Rodriguez M. Delay of gratification in children. Science. 1989;**244**(4907):933-938. DOI: 10.1126/science.2658056

[13] Rothbart MK. Temperament: A developmental framework. In: Strelau J, Angleitner A, editors. Perspectives on Individual Differences. Explorations in temperament: International perspectives on theory and measurement. 1991;**16**(4):207-212. DOI: 10.1007/978-1-4899-0643-4_5

[14] Yerkes RM, Dodson JD. The relation of strength of stimulus to rapidity of habit-formation. Journal of Comparative Neurology and Psychology. 1908;**18**(5):459-482. DOI: 10.1002/cne.920180503

[15] Tully K, Bolshakov VY. Emotional enhancement of memory: How norepinephrine enables synaptic plasticity. Molecular Brain. 2010;**3**(1):15. DOI: 10.1186/1756-6606-3-15

[16] Hamoudi A, Murray DW, Sorensen L, Fontaine A. Self-regulation and Toxic Stress: A Review of Ecological, Biological, and Developmental Studies of Self-regulation and Stress. InOPRE Report# 2015-30. Washington, DC: Office of Planning, Research and Evaluation, Administration for Children and Families, US Department of Health and Human Services; 2015

[17] Pessoa L. A network model of the emotional brain. Trends in Cognitive Sciences. 2017;**21**(5):357-371. DOI: 10.1016/j.tics.2017.03.002

[18] Banich MT. Executive Function. Current Directions in Psychological Science. 2009;**18**(2):89-94. DOI: 10.1111/j.1467-8721.2009.01615.x

[19] Banich MT, Depue BE. Recent advances in understanding neural systems that support inhibitory control. Current Opinion in Behavioral Sciences. 2015;**1**:17-22. DOI: 10.1016/j.cobeha.2014.07.006

[20] Diekhof EK, Geier K, Falkai P, Gruber O. Fear is only as deep as the mind allows. NeuroImage. 2011;**58**(1):275-285. DOI: 10.1016/j.neuroimage.2011.05.073

[21] Wierenga LM, Heuvel MPVD, Dijk SV, Rijks Y, Reus MAD, Durston S. The development of brain network architecture. Human Brain Mapping. 2015;**37**(2):717-729. DOI: 10.1002/hbm.23062

[22] McEwen BS. Brain on stress: How the social environment gets under the skin. Proceedings of the National Academy of Sciences. 2012;**109**(Supplement_2):17180-17185. DOI: 10.1073/pnas.1121254109

[23] Liston C, Miller MM, Goldwater DS, et al. Stress-induced alterations in prefrontal cortical dendritic morphology predict selective impairments in perceptual attentional set-shifting. Journal of Neuroscience. 2006;**26**(30):7870-7874. DOI: 10.1523/jneurosci.1184-06.2006

[24] Liston C, McEwen BS, Casey BJ. Psychosocial stress reversibly disrupts prefrontal processing and attentional control. Proceedings of the National Academy of Sciences of the United States of America. 2009;**106**(3):912-917. DOI: 10.1073/pnas.0807041106

[25] Dias-Ferreira E et al. Chronic stress causes frontostriatal reorganization and affects decision-making. Science. 2009;**325**:621-625

[26] Fox SE, Levitt P, Iii CAN. How the timing and quality of early experiences influence the development of brain architecture. Child Development. 2010;**81**(1):28-40. DOI: 10.1111/j.1467-8624.2009.01380.x

[27] Heim C. Psychobiological consequences of child maltreatment. In: Noll JG, Shalev I, editors. The Biology of Early Life Stress: Understanding Child Maltreatment and Trauma (15-30); Child Maltreatment Solutions Network. Switzerland: Springer International; 2018

[28] Teicher MH, Samson JA. Annual research review: Enduring neurobiological effects of childhood abuse and neglect. Journal of Child Psychology and Psychiatry. 2016;**57**(3):241-266. DOI: 10.1111/jcpp.12507

[29] Ursin H, Olff M. Psychobiology of coping and defence strategies. Neuropsychobiology. 1993;**28**(1-2):66-71. DOI: 10.1159/000119002

[30] Shonkoff JP, Garner AS, Siegel BS, et al. The lifelong effects of early childhood adversity and toxic stress. Pediatrics. 2011;**129**(1). DOI: 10.1542/peds.2011-2663

[31] Lovallo WR. Early life adversity reduces stress reactivity and enhances impulsive behavior: Implications for health behaviors. International Journal of Psychophysiology. 2013;**90**(1):8-16. DOI: 10.1016/j.ijpsycho.2012.10.006

[32] Pears KC, Fisher PA, Bruce J, Kim HK, Yoerger K. Early elementary school adjustment of maltreated children in foster care: The roles of inhibitory control and caregiver involvement. Child Development. 2010;**81**(5):1550-1564. DOI: 10.1111/j.1467-8624.2010.01491.x

[33] Cichetti D. Developmental psychopathology. In: Lamb M, Freund A, editors. The Handbook of Life-Span Development. Hoboken, NJ: Wiley; 2010. DOI: 10.1002/9780470880166.hlsd002014

[34] Welsh MC, Peterson E, Jameson MM. History of childhood maltreatment and college academic outcomes: Indirect effects of hot execution function. Frontiers in Psychology. 2017;**8**:1-13. DOI: 10.3389/fpsyg.2017.01091

[35] Welsh M, Barry PG, Jacobs AA, Beddes LA. Homeless men living in transitional housing: The BrainWise program and improvements in executive functions and coping self-efficacy. SAGE Open. 2018;**8**(2):215824401876913. DOI: 10.1177/2158244018769138

[36] Poverty Facts. Poverty Solutions. Available from: https://poverty.umich.edu/about/poverty-facts/ [Accessed: 06 June 2019]

[37] Heberle AE, Carter AS. Cognitive aspects of young children's experience of economic disadvantage. Psychological Bulletin. 2015;**141**(4):723-746. DOI: 10.1037/bul0000010

[38] Sektnan M, McClelland MM, Acock A, Morrison FJ. Relations between early family risk, childrens behavioral regulation, and academic achievement. Early Childhood Research Quarterly. 2010;**25**(4):464-479. DOI: 10.1016/j.ecresq.2010.02.005

[39] Wanless SB, McClelland MM, Tominey SL, Acock AC. The influence of demographic risk factors on childrens behavioral regulation in prekindergarten and kindergarten. Early Education and Development. 2011;**22**(3):461-488. DOI: 10.1080/10409289.2011.536132

[40] Pacheco D, Owen M, Caughy M. Growth in inhibitory control among low-income, ethnic-minority preschoolers: A group-based modeling approach. Early Childhood Research Quarterly. 2018;**42**:247-255. DOI: 10.1016/j.ecresq.2017.10.010

[41] Son S-HC, Choi JY, Kwon K-A. Reciprocal associations between inhibitory control and early academic skills: Evidence from a nationally representative sample of head start children. Early Education and Development. 2019;**30**(4):456-477. DOI: 10.1080/10409289.2019.1572382

[42] Lambert HK, King KM, Monahan KC, McLaughlin KA. Differential associations of threat and deprivation with emotion regulation and cognitive control in adolescence. Development and Psychopathology. 2016;**29**(3):929-940. DOI: 10.1017/s0954579416000584

[43] Hazzouri AZA, Elfassy T, Sidney S, Jacobs D, Stable EJP, Yaffe K. Sustained economic hardship and cognitive function: The coronary artery risk development in young adults study. American Journal of Preventive Medicine. 2017;**52**(1):1-9. DOI: 10.1016/j.amepre.2016.08.009

[44] Child Abuse and Neglect Prevention|Violence Prevention|Injury Center|CDC. Centers for Disease Control and Prevention. Available from: https://www.cdc.gov/violenceprevention/childabuseandneglect [Accessed: 06 June 2019]

[45] Felitti VJ, Anda RF, Nordenberg D, et al. Relationship of childhood abuse and household dysfunction to many of the leading causes of death in adults. American Journal of Preventive Medicine. 1998;**14**(4):245-258. DOI: 10.1016/s0749-3797(98)00017-8

[46] Augusti E-M, Melinder A. Maltreatment is associated with specific impairments in executive functions: A pilot study. Journal of Traumatic Stress. 2013;**26**(6):780-783. DOI: 10.1002/jts.21860

[47] DePrince AP, Weinzierl KM, Combs MD. Executive function performance and trauma exposure in a community sample of children. Child Abuse and Neglect. 2009;**33**(6):353-361. DOI: 10.1016/j.chiabu.2008.08.002

[48] Kirke-Smith M, Henry L, Messer D. Executive functioning: Developmental consequences on adolescents with histories of maltreatment. British Journal of Developmental Psychology. 2014;**32**(3):305-319. DOI: 10.1111/bjdp.12041

[49] Vasilevski V, Tucker A. Wide-ranging cognitive deficits in adolescents following early life maltreatment. Neuropsychology. 2016;**30**(2):239-246. DOI: 10.1037/neu0000215

[50] Marshall DF, Passarotti AM, Ryan KA, et al. Deficient inhibitory control as an outcome of childhood trauma. Psychiatry Research. 2016;**235**:7-12. DOI: 10.1016/j.psychres.2015.12.013

[51] Navalta CP. Effects of childhood sexual abuse on neuropsychological and cognitive function in college women. Journal of Neuropsychiatry. 2006;**18**(1):45-53. DOI: 10.1176/appi.neuropsych.18.1.45

[52] Shin SH, Jiskrova GK, Wills TA. Childhood maltreatment and alcohol use in young adulthood: The role of self-regulation processes. Addictive Behaviors. 2019;**90**:241-249. DOI: 10.1016/j.addbeh.2018.11.006

[53] Lafavor T. Predictors of academic success in 9- to 11-year-old homeless children: The role of executive function, social competence, and emotional control. The Journal of Early Adolescence. 2017;**38**(9):1236-1264. DOI: 10.1177/0272431616678989

[54] Obradović J. Effortful control and adaptive functioning of homeless children: Variable-focused and person-focused analyses. Journal of Applied Developmental Psychology. 2010;**31**(2):109-117. DOI: 10.1016/j.appdev.2009.09.004

[55] Schmitt SA, Finders JK, McClelland MM. Residential mobility, inhibitory control, and academic achievement in preschool. Early Education and Development. 2014;**26**(2):189-208. DOI: 10.1080/10409289.2015.975033

[56] Arnsten AF. The biology of being frazzled. Science (New York, N.Y.). 1998;**280**(5370):1711-1712

[57] Campbell WK, Krusemark EA, Dyckman KA, et al. A magnetoe-ncephalography investigation of neural correlates for social exclusion and self-control. Social Neuroscience. 2006;**1**(2):124-134

[58] Baumeister RF, Twenge JM, Nuss CK. Effects of social exclusion on cognitive processes: Anticipated aloneness reduces intelligent thought. Journal of Personality and Social Psychology. 2002;**83**(4):817-827

[59] Barnes ME, Gozal D, Molfese DL. Attention in children with obstructive sleep apnoea: An event-related potentials study. Sleep Medicine. 2012;**13**(4):368-377

[60] Tun PA, Miller-Martinez D, Lachman ME, et al. Social strain and executive function across the lifespan: The dark (and light) sides of social engagement. Neuropsychology, Development, and Cognition Section B, Aging, Neuropsychology and Cognition. 2013;**20**(3):320-338

[61] Hurstak E, Johnson JK, Tieu L, et al. Factors associated with cognitive impairment in a cohort of older homeless adults: Results from the HOPE HOME study. Drug and Alcohol Dependence. 2017;**178**:562-570

[62] Pluck G, Nakakarumai M, Sato Y. Homelessness and cognitive impairment: An exploratory study in Tokyo, Japan. East Asian Archives of Psychiatry. 2015;**25**(3):122-127

[63] Gabrielian S, Bromley E, Hamilton AB, Vu VT, Alexandrino A, et al. Problem solving skills and deficits among homeless veterans with serious mental illness. The American Journal of Orthopsychiatry. 2019;**89**(2):287-295. DOI: 10.1037/ort0000340

[64] Schutt RK, Seidman LJ, Caplan B, et al. The role of neurocognition and social context in predicting community functioning among formerly homeless seriously mentally ill persons. Schizophrenia Bulletin. 2007;**33**(6):1388-1396

[65] Essau C, LeBlanc S, llendick T. Emotion Regulation and Psychhopathology in Children and Adolescents. Oxford, UK: Oxford University Press; 2019

[66] MacLean A. The things they carry. American Sociological Review. 2010;**75**(4):563-585. DOI: 10.1177/0003122410374085

[67] Weissman JD, Russell D, Harris R, Dixon L, Haghighi F, Goodman M. Sociodemographic risk factors for serious psychological distress among U.S. veterans: Findings from the 2016 National Health Interview Survey. Psychiatric Quarterly. 2019;**90**:1-14. DOI: 10.1007/s11126-019-09651-2

[68] Sonuga-Barke EJS, Cortese S, Fairchild G, Stringaris A. Annual research review: Transdiagnostic neuroscience of child and adolescent mental disorders - differentiating decision making in attention-deficit/ hyperactivity disorder, conduct disorder, depression, and anxiety. Journal of Child Psychology and Psychiatry. 2015;**57**(3):321-349. DOI: 10.1111/jcpp.12496

[69] Wright L, Lipszyc J, Dupuis A, Thayapararajah SW, Schachar R. Response inhibition and psychopathology: A meta-analysis of go/no-go task performance. Journal of Abnormal Psychology. 2014;**123**(2):429-439. DOI: 10.1037/a0036295

[70] Braff DL, Heaton R, Kuck J, et al. The generalized pattern of neuropsychological deficits in outpatients with chronic schizophrenia with heterogeneous Wisconsin Card Sorting Test results. Archives of General Psychiatry. 1991;**48**(10):891-898

[71] Goldberg TE, Saint-Cyr JA, Weinberger DR. Assessment of procedural learning and problem solving in schizophrenic patients by Tower of Hanoi type tasks. The Journal of Neuropsychiatry and Clinical Neurosciences. 1990;**2**(2):165-173

[72] Sharma T, Antonova L. Cognitive function in schizophrenia. Deficits, functional consequences, and future treatment. Psychiatric Clinics of North America. 2003;**26**(1):25-40

[73] Crocker LD, Jurick SM, Thomas KR, et al. Worse baseline executive functioning is associated with dropout and poorer response to trauma-focused treatment for veterans with PTSD and comorbid traumatic brain injury. Behaviour Research and Therapy. 2018;**108**:68-77

[74] Knight MJ, Baune BT. Executive function and spatial cognition mediate psychosocial dysfunction in major depressive disorder. Frontiers in Psychiatry. 2018;**9**:539

[75] Insel TR, Fernald RD. How the brain processes social information: Searching for the social brain. Annual Review of Neuroscience. 2004;**27**(1):697-722. DOI: 10.1146/annurev.neuro.27.070203.144148

[76] Sapolsky RM. Behave: The Biology of Humans at our Best and Worst. 5th ed. New York: Penguin; 2017. 800p

[77] Sloboda Z, Petras H, Robertson E. Prevention of substance use. In: Hingson R, editor. Switzerland: Springer; 2019

[78] Kandel ER. Neuroscience: Breaking down scientific barriers to the study of brain and mind. Science. 2000;**290**(5494):1113-1120. DOI: 10.1126/science.290.5494.1113

[79] Pennington BF, Ozonoff S. Executive functions and developmental psychopathology. Journal of Child Psychology and Psychiatry. 1996;**37**(1):51-87. DOI: 10.1111/j.1469-7610.1996.tb01380.x

[80] Welsh MC, Pennington BF, Groisser DB. A normative-developmental study of executive function: A window on prefrontal function in children. Developmental Neuropsychology. 1991;**7**(2):131-149. DOI: 10.1080/87565649109540483

[81] Luria A. The frontal lobes and the regulation of behavior. Psychophysiology of the Frontal Lobes. 1973:3-26. DOI: 10.1016/b978-0-12-564340-5.50006-8

[82] Llorens-Martín M. Exercising new neurons to vanquish Alzheimer disease. Brain Plasticity. 2018;**4**(1):111-126. DOI: 10.3233/bpl-180065

[83] Kishiyama MM, Boyce WT, Jimenez AM, Perry LM, Knight RT. Sociodemographic disparities affect prefrontal function in children. Journal of Cognitive Neuroscience. 2008;**21**:1106-1115. DOI: 10.1162/jocn.2009.21101

[84] Schilling EA, Aseltine RH, Gore S. Adverse childhood experiences and mental health in young adults: A longitudinal survey. BMC Public Health. 2007;**7**(1):30-40. DOI: 10.1186/1471-2458-7-30

[85] Durlak JA, Weissberg RP, Dymnicki AB, Taylor RD, Schellinger KB. The impact of enhancing students' social and emotional learning: A meta-analysis of school-based universal interventions. Child Development. 2011;**82**(1):405-432. DOI: 10.1111/j.1467-8624.2010.01564.x

[86] McClelland M, Geldhof J, Morrison F, Gestsdottir S, Camerson C, Bowers E, et al. Self-regulation. In: Halfon N, Forrest C, Lerner R, Faustman E, editors. Handbook of Life Course Health Development. Switzerland: Springer; 2018. p. 275-298

[87] Insel T. From neurons to neighborhoods: Charting a new science of mental health. Wu Tsai Neuroscience Institute, Stanford University; October 2014

[88] Center on the Developing Child at Harvard University. Available from: https://developingchild.harvard.edu/ [Accessed: 06 June 2019]

[89] Teaster PB, Stansbury KL, Nerenberg L, Stanis P. An adult

protective services' view of collaboration with mental health services. Journal of Elder Abuse & Neglect. 2009;**21**(4):289-306. DOI: 10.1080/08946560903004821

[90] Dusenbury L. A review of research on fidelity of implementation: Implications for drug abuse prevention in school settings. Health Education Research. 2003;**18**(2):237-256. DOI: 10.1093/her/18.2.237

[91] Escoffery C, Lebow-Skelley E, Udelson H, et al. A scoping study of frameworks for adapting public health evidence-based interventions. Translational Behavioral Medicine. 2018;**9**(1):1-10. DOI: 10.1093/tbm/ibx067

[92] Brabeck M, Jeffrey J, Fry S. Practice for knowledge acquisition (not drill and kill). https://www.apa.org/education/K12/p

[93] Connell JP. A new multidimensional measure of childrens perceptions of control. Child Development. 1985;**56**(4):1018. DOI: 10.2307/1130113

[94] Custers EJFN. Long-term retention of basic science knowledge: A review study. Advances in Health Sciences Education. 2010;**15**(1):109-128. DOI: 10.1007/s10459-008-9101-y

[95] Barry PG, Welsh M. The BrainWise curriculum: Neurocognitive development intervention Program. In: Romer D, Walker EF, editors. Adolescent psychopathology and the Developing Brain: Integrating Brain and Prevention Sciene. NY: Oxford University press. pp. 420-440. ISBN: 978-0-19-530625-5

[96] A Proven Evidence-based Approach. The BrainWise Program. Available from: https://www.brainwise-plc.org/ [Accessed: 06 June 2019]

[97] History. The BrainWise Program. Available from: https://www.brainwise-plc.org/about/history/ [Accessed: 06 June 2019]

[98] Ledoux J. Fear and the brain: Where have we been, and where are we going? Biological Psychiatry. 1998;**44**(12):1229-1238. DOI: 10.1016/s0006-3223(98)00282-0

[99] Riggs NR, Greenberg MT, Kusché CA, Pentz MA. The mediational role of neurocognition in the behavioral outcomes of a social-emotional prevention program in elementary school students: Effects of the PATHS curriculum. Prevention Science. 2006;**7**(1):91-102. DOI: 10.1007/s11121-005-0022-1

[100] Cacioppo S, Grippo AJ, London S, Goossens L, Cacioppo JT. Loneliness. Perspectives on Psychological Science. 2015;**10**(2):238-249. DOI: 10.1177/1745691615570616

[101] Cyranowski JM, Zill N, Bode R, et al. Assessing social support, companionship, and distress: National Institute of Health (NIH) Toolbox Adult Social Relationship Scales. Health Psychology. 2013;**32**(3):293-301. DOI: 10.1037/a0028586

[102] Southwick SM, Morgan CA, Vythilingam M, Charney D. Mentors enhance resilience in at-risk children and adolescents. Psychoanalytic Inquiry. 2007;**26**(4):577-584. DOI: 10.1080/07351690701310631

[103] Holt-Lunstad J, Robles TF, Sbarra DA. Advancing social connection as a public health priority in the United States. American Psychologist. 2017;**72**(6):517-530. DOI: 10.1037/amp0000103

[104] Donahue MJ, Benson PL. Religion and the well-being of adolescents. Journal of Social Issues. 1995;**51**(2):145-160. DOI: 10.1111/j.1540-4560.1995.tb01328.x

[105] Southwick SM, Vythilingam M, Charney DS. The psychobiology of depression and resilience to stress: Implications for prevention and treatment. Annual Review of

Clinical Psychology. 2005;**1**(1):255-291. DOI: 10.1146/annurev.clinpsy.1.102803.143948

[106] Diamond A, Lee K. Interventions shown to aid executive function development in children 4 to 12 years old. Science. 2011;**333**(6045):959-964. DOI: 10.1126/science.1204529

[107] Ericson KM, Laibson D. Intertemporal choice. National Bureau of Economic Research (NBER) Working Paper No. 25358. December 2018. http://www.nber.org/papers/w25358

[108] Parkinson RG. The common cause: Creating race and nation in the american revolution. Chapel Hill: University of North Carolina Press; 768 p

[109] McGrew S, Ortega, T, Breaksonte J, Wineburg S. The challenge that's bigger than fake news: Civic reasoning in a social media environment. American Educator. 2017;Fall:4-10

[110] Wineberg J, Mann S. Salford Jewish Community Health Research Report 2015. Available from: https://archive.jpr.org.uk/object-uk370 (Published January 1, 1970) [Accessed: 06 June 2019]

[111] Naifeh JA, Nock MK, Ursano RJ, Vegella PL, Aliaga PA, et al. Neurocognitive function and suicidal behavior in US Army soldiers. Suicide Life Threat Behavior. 2017;**47**(5):589-602. DOI: 10.1111/SLTB.12307

[112] Marteau TM, Hollands GJ, Fletcher PC. Changing human behavior to prevent disease: The importance of targeting automatic processes. Science. 2012;**337**(6101):1492-1495. DOI: 10.1126/science.1226918

[113] Barry P. Research and Results. The BrainWise Program. Available from: https://www.brainwise-plc.org/research-results/ [Accessed: 06 June 2019]

[114] Norwood S, Rosa J, Fairbanks K, Downes D, Cerbana C, Gorman Barry P. Promoting the development of executive functioning for children from 1st through 5th grade using BrainWise. In: Poster Presented at the Rocky Mounting Psychological Association Conference; Boise, ID; 2015

[115] Persing R, Gorman Barry P, Welsh M, Cazzell K, Peifer, Reyes A. Improving health decisions in atrisk families: Nurse home visits, BrainWise and technology. In: Poster presented at the Colorado Public Health Association Conference; Pueblo, CO; 2011

[116] Bousman CA, Twamley EW, Vella L, et al. Homelessness and neuropsychological Impairment. The Journal of Nervous and Mental Disease. 2010;**198**(11):790-794. DOI: 10.1097/nmd.0b013e3181f97dff

[117] Henry M, Mahathey A, Morrill T, Robinson A, Shivji A, Watt R, et al. The 2018 Annual Homeless Assessment Report (AHAR) to Congress. Washington, D.C.: U.S. Department of Housing and Urban Health Office of Community Planning and Development; 2018

[118] O'Connell M, Kasprow W, Rosenheck RA. National dissemination of supported housing in the VA: Model adherence versus model modification. Psychiatric Rehabilitation Journal. 2010;**33**(4):308-319

[119] Tsai J, Rosenheck RA. Risk factors for homelessness among US veterans. Epidemiologic Reviews. 2015;**37**:177-195

[120] Wenzel SL et al. Indicators of chronic homelessness among veterans. Hospital & Community Psychiatry. 1993;**44**(12):1172-1176

[121] Goldfinger SM, Schutt RK, Tolomiczenko GS, Seidman L, Penk WE, Turner W, et al. Housing

placement and subsequent days homeless among formerly homeless adults with mental illness. Psychiatric Services. 1999;**50**(5):674-679

[122] Palermo S. Crossing in the red zone: mTBI/concussion in the context of war. EC Psychology and Psychiatry. 2018;**7**:287-288

[123] Woon FL, Farrer TJ, Braman CR, Mabey JK, Hedges DW. A meta-analysis of the relationship between symptom severity of posttraumatic stress disorder and executive function. Cognitive Neuropsychiatry. 2016;**22**(1):1-16. DOI: 10.1080/13546805.2016.1255603

[124] MacDonald BC, Flashman LA, Saykin AJ. Executive dysfunction following traumatic brain injury: Neural substrates and treatment strategies. NeuroRehabilitation. 2002;**17**:333-344

[125] Rabinowitz AR, Levin HS. Cognitive sequelae of traumatic brain injury. Psychiatric Clinics of North America. 2014;**37**(1):1-11. DOI: 10.1016/j.psc.2013.11.004

[126] Newcombe VFJ, Outtrim JG, Chatfield DA, et al. Parcellating the neuroanatomical basis of impaired decision-making in traumatic brain injury. Brain. 2011;**134**(3):759-768. DOI: 10.1093/brain/awq388

[127] Simmons MM, Gabrielian S, Byrne T, McCullough MB, Smith JL, Taylor TJ, et al. A hybrid III stepped wedge cluster randomized trial testing an implementation strategy to facilitate the use of an evidence-based practice in VA Homeless Primary Care Treatment Programs. Implementation Science. 2017;**12**(1):46-55

Chapter 6

When Aggression Is Out of Control: From One-Person to Two-Person Neuropsychology

J. Gagnon, J.E. Quansah and W.S. Kim

Abstract

From a neuropsychological perspective, impulsive aggression and its treatment are usually conceptualized in most research as a closed executive functioning system, as though the behavior was the product of the person's cerebral functioning only. However, recent studies in social cognitive neuroscience have emphasized the influence of social factors on cognitive processes and cerebral functioning for the development and maintenance of impulsive aggression. This chapter will review studies that highlight the relevance of initiating a shift of paradigm from a one-person-cerebral functioning model to a social interactive-cerebral functioning model of impulsive aggression. First, the influences of an aversive environment on a child's cognitive processes and executive functioning will be discussed with the aim of explaining the development of impulsive aggressive behaviors in early childhood. Second, we will review studies that have shown how the link between social information processes and executive/inhibitory functioning serve to maintain behaviors. Finally, strengths and weaknesses of existing inhibitory control strategies will be discussed with the intention of proposing some novel ideas that incorporate a two-person neuropsychological approach.

Keywords: impulsive aggression, executive functions, inhibitory processes, social information processing, child development, treatment, inhibitory control training, implementation intentions

1. Introduction

When facing a dangerous or threatening situation, aggression is a behavioral response that is often appropriate and necessary. An individual who is unable to perceive the hostile intentions of others is also unable to protect him- or herself or their personal needs. Aggression can also be characterized as a vital energy that allows an individual to mobilize the physical and psychological resources necessary to compete with others in a healthy way. Finally, aggression is present in many positive forms of emotional expression; it gives rise to creativity and the establishment of new relationships. It is when aggression is out of control that it becomes unbeneficial, problematic, and potentially harmful. Lack of control over the intensity, form, and timing of aggressive behavior is thus an issue of interest to clinicians who would like to help people with uncontrolled aggression.

IntechOpen

The defining characteristic of impulsive aggression is uncontrolled and impulsive behavioral manifestations of anger in response to a provocation [1]. Aggressive behaviors have a negative impact on social, legal, and health-care systems, and are significant predictors of long-term social dysfunction [2]. Consequently, understanding and preventing aggressive behavior is a worldwide major public health concern [3]. Impulsive aggression is also associated with violent forms of aggression, which often occur in the context of interpersonal relationships [4]. When considering the importance of the social dimension in models of impulsive aggression, this observation is not surprising. While many of these models have come from social psychology, contributions from neuroscience have increasingly allowed for the inclusion of the social component, with the aim to produce more integrative models. This has opened up the field and made it possible to explore how cerebral connectivity may vary according to distinct social inputs and the reaction to those inputs.

The purpose of this chapter is to reflect on new avenues of intervention that are based on *both* social psychology and neuroscience models. We believe that inhibitory control training (ICT) represents a unique opportunity by which this may happen. Indeed, ICT addresses impulse control disorders and, in this sense, may be a relevant intervention strategy for impulsive aggression. However, to adapt it to the peculiarities of impulsive aggression, one must proceed with careful deliberation. It is here that our analogy with two-person psychology comes into play. The term "two-person psychology" comes from a clinical psychology approach, which means that the emotions and subjective reactions of the client and the therapist during a psychotherapy session are not only determined by the client's dynamics but also by the mental life of the therapist [5]. The personal reactions of the therapist are part of the session; they not only influence the interactional processes in the dyad [6] but they also contribute to the transformation and therapeutic change, as experienced by the client [7]. Inspired by this clinical approach, we will propose that ICT may be integrated into impulsive aggression treatment programs if it is extended into the social realm, and more particularly to social cognition. To do this, we believe that an intervention strategy called *implementation intentions* can bridge the gap between ICT and the field of social cognition.

Before discussing these methods of intervention, we will review evidence of the social determinants of aggressive impulsive behavior. We will begin by looking at the influence of aversive social environments on the development of social cognition and inhibition in children. We will then discuss how social and neurobiological models can shed light on the factors that maintain aggression in adults.

2. Development of hostile cognitive structures in early childhood

Aversive early childhood experiences and environments, which include physical or psychological abuse, inconsistent or severe discipline, parental neglect, social rejection, exposure to aggressive peers or violence, among many others, have all been identified in the literature as constituting important risk factors of disruptive and aggressive behavioral problems later in life [8–10]. Here, we will present some of the evidence-based theories that explain how early life social adversity affects the development of a child's mental processes and is believed to increase the likelihood of future aggressive behavior.

2.1 Social cognition and the influence of aversive childhood environments

In cognitive psychology, social information processing (SIP) models postulate that in a person's memory, there exists a collection of memories of past experiences.

In this pool of memories, accumulated information is thought to bind together, forming stable structures of concepts and sets of principles. These organized sets are often called schemas, and they guide a person's behavior in social situations [11, 12]. An individual who was physically abused as a child may have an accumulation of aggressive social experiences stored in memory. Over time, aggressive thought and belief patterns may develop and lead to aggressive behavior.

A *schema* (also referred to as a "script"; [13]) can be described as a network of associative concepts that are stored in memory and function to organize past experiences—to make sense of the world and absorb new knowledge efficiently [14, 15].

Imagine a person is approaching you with a big smile and a hand raised up high. If you have had past experiences of giving someone a "high five," then it is likely that the smile and the raised hand (which are "encoded" in the current situation) will be interpreted as a friendly gesture. Given past experiences, it is unlikely that you will assume they have harmful intentions. Now, let us imagine that this person is someone with whom you would like to become friends. You remember that past occurrences of returning a "high five" have helped you attain a similar goal with other people. This cognitive process leads you to decide to gently tap the person's hand "up high." From a cognitive psychology perspective, the schema in this situation contains concepts such as a "smile," a "raised hand," a "high five," a "non-harmful intention," a "friendship," and a "positive experience," and these concepts are associated together with past experiences.

Now, this time try to imagine the same situation, but as it might happen with a child who has experienced physical abuse. The schema evoked here would likely be quite different. It may contain concepts such as a "smile," a "raised hand," a "slap on the face," a "harmful intention," a "threat," or a "negative experience." While the initial situation—a person approaches with a big smile and a raised hand—is the same in both examples, it is unlikely that the child who was abused would react, or behave, in the same manner as in the situation above.

2.2 Schemas biased toward hostility

While a schema can be a cognitive structure that helps process social information efficiently, it can also omit details and induce errors. Because schemas are formed by past experiences, recurrent negative events and early aversive experiences may influence certain schemas in such a way that they become biased. As a result, a person may be misled by their interpretations and react with aggressive behavior. For example, what if the child mentioned above had decided to hit the person in order to run away. Had the person who approached the child been intending to cause harm, then the child's aggressive behavior would have potentially helped them avoid a slap on the face. However, if the child repeatedly uses this schema and reacts aggressively in every social situation, then this will result in a chronic accessibility of hostile schemas [16, 17] and a frequent hostile interpretation of the behavior of others (hostile attribution bias; [11, 18, 19]).

2.3 Schema formation through observation

Research evidence on early exposure to media violence (as depicted on television [TV], movies, video games, cell phones, online/computer sources, etc.) has shown that hostile schemas formed in childhood do not *only* develop from direct exposure to aggression (e.g., actual physical or verbal abuse). They can also result from *indirect* exposure—through the observation of aggressive acts as depicted by individuals in violent media [12, 20, 21]. Because a schema acts as an associative network of concepts, a stimulus may activate a concept, which then activates other associated concepts that are part of the same network. In this way, a schema can be implicitly activated (or "primed") by a stimulus and trigger a chain-like reaction between associated concepts within a particular network [22, 23]. It is important to note, however, that there is a difference between schemas that occur during adulthood, and those that develop earlier in life. Adults often have schemas that were acquired through accumulated experiences, and this serves to strengthen the links between associated concepts, making them highly resistant to change. By contrast, a child's schemas are much more flexible and impressionable, making it much easier to encode new information. While this is a key component that contributes to social learning, it can also make children more vulnerable when exposed to aggressive stimuli [24]. A child who observes a violent scene on TV will encode aggressive cues without difficulty, and often without filter. The more the child is exposed to such media violence, the more the links between concepts of aggression will be reinforced, and these aggression-related concepts will create additional links with other concepts from memory. With frequent repetition of this process, activated aggressive schemas will expand, become chronically accessible, and resistant to change. Indeed, longitudinal studies have shown that children's early hostile schemas contribute to the stability and maintenance of later aggressive behaviors [25].

2.4 Normative beliefs

The term *normative beliefs* refers to an individual's personal standard about the appropriateness of particular social behaviors [26]. In other words, they serve to determine which behavior is appropriate versus inappropriate in a given social situation. They are distinct from social norms or *perceived* social norms, which are the *actual* social consensus on a given social behavior or the individuals' perception of the existing social consensus, respectively.

Guerra et al. proposed that normative beliefs are acquired through a socialization process, which occurs with a primary caregiver, a significant reference group, and through personal evaluation [27]. First, a child's primary caregivers play an important role for their social development and have an incredible influence, especially on infants. Caregivers or parents are the usually the first source of verbalized rules, normative beliefs, and social norms, which are quickly encoded and integrated into early childhood cognition. They also contribute to the establishment of an infant's personal normative beliefs. Second, children develop normative beliefs through social exchanges with other individuals as well, such as peers, extended family members, or a significant reference group. As a child interacts within these networks of people, they can be easily influenced and may accommodate new rules, socials norms, and beliefs. Third, children construct normative beliefs that are coherent with their own evaluative schemas. Briefly, this evaluative schema contains a response evaluation, outcome expectancies, and a self-efficacy assessment [11]. Respectively, these refer to an assessment of the quality of certain morally- and value-based social responses (e.g., morally good vs. morally bad responses), to personal opinions about the results of these responses (i.e., thoughts about the consequences of these responses within the social realm), and to the degree of confidence they have in their ability to successfully perform these behaviors and achieve a particular desired outcome (i.e., an assessment of one's capacity to successfully perform a chosen social response). It has been theorized that if a child's evaluative schema is biased toward aggression and/or hostility, then they will develop normative beliefs that approve aggressive social responses. Furthermore, these aggression-related normative beliefs are thought to crystalize over time, thus promoting an increase in aggressive behavior throughout the lifespan. Indeed, it has been found that aggressive children, as compared to their non-aggressive peers, will (1) evaluate aggressive responses more favorably [28, 29], (2) are more likely to expect a favorable outcome if physical or verbal aggression is used [30–32], and (3) feel more confident about their efficacy when performing behaviors that are physically and/or verbally aggressive [31–33].

2.5 Negative social feedbacks

There is now empirical evidence supporting the fact that environmental factors (such as witnessing acts of aggression) and emotion dysregulation (e.g., difficulty in controlling one's anger) are predicted by aggressive normative beliefs, and that these beliefs predict subsequent aggressive behavior [34]. Furthermore, children who engage in these acts of aggression may provoke aggressive tendencies in others and thus create or stimulate an aversive environment. Within this hostile atmosphere, children often exchange negative social feedback, which only serves to reinforce aggressive normative beliefs and behaviors (also referred to as a "self-fulfilling prophecy effect"). As this pattern repeats itself, it becomes of a vicious cycle of aversive environmental triggers, aggressive cognitions, and aggressive behavioral responses [35].

2.6 Executive functions and early aversive environments

Executive functions are higher order cognitive abilities that are responsible for the regulation of thoughts, emotions, and actions [36, 37]. While there are many different ways to define or describe executive functioning, it is generally thought to comprise (1) cognitive control of planning or organizing action(s), (2) monitoring a series of responses [38–40], (3) divided attention or attentional control, (4) abstract reasoning, (5) alertness, and importantly, (6) behavioral regulation or inhibition [41–43]. A recent study that used a behavioral assessment of reactive aggressive behavior (i.e., an emotion-driven impulsive act in response to a perceived threat) found that the degree to which a participant could inhibit their responses (also known in cognitive psychology as "response inhibition") was the strongest predictor of reactive aggression. This finding held when compared to other cognitive processes such as working memory, cognitive flexibility, and attentional control [43, 44]. For this reason, when examining early childhood factors that play a role in the development of aggressive behavior, we have placed an important focus on cognitive processes that relate to inhibition.

As previously mentioned, inhibition is an executive function that allows a person to inhibit a dominant response [45]. It has primarily been linked to brain function involving the prefrontal cortex (PFC). Many neurocognitive researchers have shown that child maltreatment can affect specific brain regions within fronto-limbic networks [46–50]. The implicated brain regions include the PFC, the orbitofrontal cortex, the anterior cingular cortex, and the amygdala [46, 48, 50, 51]. According to the "Interactive Specialization model" by Johnson [52], some cortical regions, which are responsible for neuronal maturation and specialization, become functionally efficient by having sufficient neural activation. It is possible that maltreatment in infancy disturbs these activations. Also, increased density of glucocorticoid receptors due to early life stress (such as maltreatment in infancy) is theorized to negatively affect the early maturation of the PFC [53].

2.7 Inhibition and the social environment

Numerous studies have demonstrated that impaired inhibitory control interacts with the cognitive functions involved in processing social information. More specifically, both the interpretation and response decision steps have been linked to deficits in inhibitory control, which predicts aggressive behavior [54–58]. Difficulties in inhibiting hostile schemas may lead children to habitually interpret others' behavior as being hostile (hostile attribution bias), and low inhibitory control increases the probability of choosing the most salient and dominant response (e.g., behavioral aggression).

From an evolutionary-developmental perspective, low inhibitory control is not necessarily considered as an impairment in cognitive function, but rather a form of adaptation amidst an unstable environment [59, 60]. For example, one study found that individuals who grow up in harsh and unpredictable environments (e.g., dangerous, crime-ridden neighborhoods) prefer smaller immediate rewards over larger future rewards [61]. In other words, within dangerous and unstable environments, a preference for immediate rewards may be more adaptive than a preference for delayed rewards in an uncertain future [62]. From this perspective, inhibition would be an inefficient function, as it prevents people from taking advantage of immediate benefits [63]. Therefore, it is possible that early childhood adversity decreases inhibitory control in order to help a child better adapt to particular environments, which may explain the relationship between low inhibitory control, uninhibited aggressive behaviors, and early adverse social experiences.

Taken together, a solid literature links early social adversity in childhood to aggression, and this happens through socio-cognitive mediators such as aggressive schemas, normative beliefs that support aggression, and low inhibitory control. It is important to note, however, that childhood adversity is one of *many* risk factors related to aggressive behavior, and adverse social experiences in early age does not necessarily lead to aggressive behavior in adulthood. In the following section, we will discuss other contributing social factors, how they interact with cognitive and neurobiological function, and how they may serve to maintain aggressive behavior over time.

3. Underlying factors that perpetuate impulsive aggression in adulthood

3.1 The neural substrates of impulsive aggression

In most social contexts, even those involving a conflict or altercation, an impulsively aggressive act can result in unnecessary harm, serious injury, and even death [64, 65]. Having the ability to implement and execute context-appropriate regulation strategies will play an important role in shaping how a person will react to stressors or unpredictable situations later in life. As previously mentioned, human neuro-behavioral functioning is not *solely* influenced by early-life situational factors. *Individual differences* in genetic disposition, cognitive ability and flexibility, emotion regulation, and behavioral inhibition, as well as many other internal and external factors, will all have major implications for a person's capacity to have healthy and adaptive interactions within the social realm.

3.2 The effects of cortical and subcortical neural imbalance

Much of what we presently know regarding the brain-behavior dynamics of impulsive aggression was acquired from examining case studies of individuals who suffered from brain trauma, neural lesions, or brain tissue damage due to illness or disease [39]. A well-known example is that of Phineas Gage, a nineteenth century railroad worker who survived a horrific accident whereby a large iron rod pierced through his skull, destroying a large portion of his left frontal lobe. While this tragedy resulted in deleterious effects on his personality, social relationships and general quality of life, it also served to enable ground-breaking discoveries in the domain of neural specialization and functionality. In particular, the area damaged during the accident—the PFC—was subsequently linked to the regulation of emotional states such as anger and impulsivity, as well as maladaptive behaviors, like impulsive aggression [66].

Researchers examining the link between PFC function (or cortical regions, more generally) and impulsive aggression have looked at various components of cognitive processes such as *executive functioning*. Furthermore, neurochemical imbalances in the level of the steroid hormones cortisol and testosterone, as well as fluctuations in the modulation of neurotransmitters such as serotonin, have all been shown to induce physiological changes in core affective and cognitive processing brain regions, which have an important influence on the way an individual perceives and acts in response to social threats [67].

3.3 Dysregulation of social behavior networks

The tendency to habitually respond to a perceived threat in an aggressive manner is not governed by frontal brain regions alone; rather, it is thought to be maintained by a complex interplay of cognitive, affective, and behavioral neural systems [39, 68]. Researchers examining these mechanisms in relation to impulsive aggressive urges and behaviors have proposed that a disruption in decision-making and social-emotional information processing circuits is also a key contributor [39]. From a cognitive neuroscience approach, it is posited that an imbalance in top-down control (primarily governed by prefrontal brain regions) and activity in subcortical areas responsible for "bottom-up" processes (i.e., "feed-forward" modulation of emotional, appetitive, as well as aggressive reactivity) leads to difficulties in behavioral inhibition [68]. Abnormal activation in fronto-parietal regions may enhance impulsive drives, such as the urge to respond aggressively to a social provocation [65, 69]. For example, in an examination of aggressive behavior in relation to frontal-lobe functioning, Giancola and Zeichner used neuropsychological measures to test young men in a social-provocation paradigm [42]. Results indicated that men who performed poorly on the tests were significantly more aggressive toward peers, as compared to those who performed better. The researchers proposed the possibility that diminished frontal-lobe functioning coupled with provoking external conditions (e.g., social provocation) may lead to decreases in behavioral inhibition and a heightening of aggressive reactivity [42]. This finding is further validated by studies examining specific cognitive impairments linked to recurrent antisocial behavior and the tendency to reoffend in criminal populations (i.e., recidivism). A recent meta-analysis concluded that impairments in inhibition—the executive function that is particularly important for behavioral self-regulation and the suppression of dominant impulses—were a significant predictor of future acts of physical aggression and violent crime [70].

Researchers have also used functional magnetic resonance imaging (fMRI) to examine neural activity within the social behavior network in real time (i.e., in vivo). Numerous studies have replicated evidence of critical interconnections between frontal cortices, subcortical regions, and striatal brain regions in the maintenance of aggressive response patterns (for review, see [71]). The flow of activity within these connections regulates emotional processing, which acts to modulate behavioral reactivity [72, 73]. For example, in an fMRI study by Coccaro and colleagues, brain regions that have previously been linked to impulsive aggression were assessed for functional deficits [74]. Results indicated that individuals with high aggressivity (as compared to healthy controls) showed greater activation in the amygdala—a subcortical brain structure thought to play a key role in emotional processing, threat detection, and in activating stress-induced behavioral response [74–76]. Inversely, healthy controls showed greater activation in frontal regions when viewing the emotional faces [74]. Similarly, Nomura [77] found that healthy participants who viewed emotional images showed an inverse functional connectivity between the amygdala and brain regions thought to be responsible for integrating affective information, emotional valuation, and decision-making processes. By contrast, individuals who met criteria for intermittent explosive disorder (a psychiatric disorder characterized by emotional dysregulation and pathological impulsive aggression) failed to show such functional connectivity [71, 77]. The results suggest that individuals who have difficulty regulating emotions and inhibiting aggressive impulses may have impaired connectivity in the cortico-limbic pathway [71].

3.4 The influence of emotional reactivity within the social sphere

More recently, researchers have investigated the neural substrates of impulsive aggression in relation to social situations that provoke negative emotional reactivity (e.g., feelings of anger or hostility, betrayal, jealousy, social exclusion or peer rejection; [78, 79]). In addition to the importance of past social experiences, it has been suggested that rejection is one of the *most common precursors* of aggression and one of the *most significant risk factors* for adolescent violence [79, 80]. After an incidence of social rejection, studies have shown that people fail to process situational information in an efficient and adaptive manner, which leads to reductions in self-control [81].

The question of why some individuals respond to particular social exchanges by increasing their efforts to gain acceptance or reconcile a conflict, while other individuals tend to respond with increased aggression and acts of retaliation, is an area of research that is still being explored. One such investigation, by Chester and colleagues tested whether social rejection triggered aggressive reactivity through heightened activation in areas of the brain associated with emotional pain or anger. They further assessed whether individual differences in executive functioning moderated this relationship [73]. Findings were consistent with socio-cognitive models positing that for some individuals, social rejection triggers negative emotional responses such as anger, which may lead to maladaptive cognitive appraisals and deficits in decision-making strategies, thus triggering the impulse to act aggressively [13]. Similarly, in a study that included healthy female and male participants, Achterberg and colleagues investigated aggressive feelings and behaviors in relation to negative social feedback [82]. Conjunction neuroimaging findings from the study found greater activation in the right dorsal lateral PFC during negative feedback (as compared to neutral feedback), which was significantly associated with shorter noise blasts (an index of lower levels of aggression) in response to negative evaluations from peers. The results suggest that particular areas within the PFC factor into the regulation of affective impulsive actions, such as socially provoked aggression [82].

3.5 Social information-processing mechanisms

Pioneered by developmental researchers, such as Crick and Dodge [11], major advances in our understanding of social behavior more generally have emerged from studies on social cognition and social adjustment during childhood [83–85]. Over the last few decades, the social information-processing model (SIP; [11]) has been extensively researched. It has paved the way for a better understanding of how social cognitive constructs formed early in childhood can perpetuate a cycle of maladaptive behavioral response patterns throughout the lifespan [25, 86]. Indeed, a considerable amount of evidence has supported a significant relationship between deficits or difficulties in social cognitive processing and higher levels of aggressive response patterns during social interactions [87, 88].

The general SIP model [11] (here, adapted for adults) proposes that when a person enters a social situation, they are already primed with a set of biologically determined cognitive capacities and a history of social experiences that are stored in long-term memory. Amidst an array of social cues, their ensuing behavioral response is thought to be a function of how they have processed those cues. In a sequential manner, it is hypothesized that the person begins the social interaction by selectively attending to cues on both an internal level (e.g., related to affective or cognitive processes) and external level (i.e., related to situational/environmental stimuli). After encoding the cues, the person interprets them according to a number of evaluative processes. They may filter the information in accordance to their own personalized knowledge structures (i.e., mental representations that are based on similar social scenarios from previous experiences). They may also make inferences and attribute intentions to the person(s) involved in the interaction, and evaluate how they handled similar social exchanges in the past. Next, they determine whether or not the strategies they used in the past were successful in achieving the goal(s) that they had set out to obtain. Depending on how they perceive their self-efficacy (i.e., self-assessment of past performance) and the degree to which they deem past strategies successful, they form predictions or expectations about the outcome of using a similar strategy in the current situation [11].

After interpreting the situation, the person then proceeds by clarifying their goals, while taking into consideration their desired outcome (e.g., settling a previous dispute, taking revenge for a past offense, asserting a sense of control or power, etc.). This evaluation is thought to be highly influenced by the person's present state of arousal, which acts to orientate them toward achieving their goal. It is also at this step that a person may revise their goals or find different strategies that may be more appropriate to the current situation. In some circumstances, a quick response is necessary and it may be more feasible to construct a new response strategy or re-adjust their outcome expectations. According to the SIP model, once a response has been selected, the behavioral enactment ensues. However, a person may have difficulty or deficits in regulating the intensity of their affective arousal. If the person is unable or unwilling to select or produce an adaptive response, then it is likely that impulsive urges will interrupt the decision-making process and cognitive control mechanisms. As is often the case with impulsive aggressive acts, when a breakdown in inhibitory control occurs, withholding a potentially maladaptive response may prove to be difficult or unattainable [89].

3.6 Integrating information-processing theories with complex dynamical models

When factoring in that many social interactions involve a number of uncertainties and ambiguities (e.g., knowledge of the motivations or perceptions of the other parties involved), it can be challenging to quickly process, generate, refine, and select an appropriate behavioral response. For this reason, many information-processing (IP) models have been criticized for the rigidity of their linear structure and lack of complexity in explaining *actual* brain function and activity (e.g., mechanistic explanations of dynamic neural systems, contingent features, nonlinear connectivity as it happens in *real time*, etc.; [11]). Despite these shortcomings, IP paradigms clearly have a heuristic value and one of the most effective applications of their principles are in providing a basic understanding of how active social cognitive processes may contribute to emotional and behavioral reactivity.

Since its original conception, the SIP model has been reformulated to reflect a more complex, cyclical process, whereby multiple cognitive processes may occur simultaneously and operate in a time-related sequence [11]. Some reformulated IP models have made the distinction between information that is processed "online" (working representations gathered from the immediate environment) and information that is processed "offline" (knowledge structures stored in long-term memory; [25]). The online representations are hypothesized to contain information from social cues that are encoded during the onset of interaction. Here, particular emotionally charged cues may evoke attentional biases that facilitate hostile attributions [90]. In situations where missing or ambiguous environmental data occur, online representations are thought to be supplemented or "filled in" by information taken from stored knowledge structures [25].

This revised formulation demonstrates how *active* cognitive processes can be *directly* influenced by previous social interactions. With repetition, these processes may be conditioned over time, and thus serve as a control mechanism for a variety of impulsive behaviors [11, 91, 92]. Indeed, if a person regularly evokes a particular knowledge structure (e.g., "Social encounters are inherently hostile"), then "offline" information (e.g., "When someone gives me a dirty look, it means I need to watch my back") may repeatedly find its way into a person's "online" representations ("They're giving me *that look*. I won't let them be the first to attack").

Notably, personal motivations and expectations regarding social interaction are multi-factorial. Furthermore, a person's baseline affect (i.e., their current emotional state) will play a critical role, both in *how* the person is likely to interpret a particular social situation and *what* they are likely to "select" as a response. Despite the multitude of factors that may contribute to the maintenance of impulsive aggression, one of the primary goals of this chapter is to examine and integrate evidence-based knowledge on the control mechanisms involved so that a better understanding may facilitate effective interventions.

4. Adaptation of inhibitory-control training in the treatment of impulsive aggression

Although an impulsive response that is aggressive in nature may appear on the surface as a simple disinhibited reaction to an internal or external trigger, the studies reviewed in the previous sections invite us to develop a conception of impulsive aggression that is much wider. Here, we underline *the person* as being in constant interaction with his or her social environment during the selection, or lack thereof, of his or her behavioral responses. It is during his or her social interactions that all the active social cognitive processes which underlie aggressive behaviors are being played out. In addition, early interactions experienced in childhood are gradually transformed into cognitive structures (e.g., hostile schemas or aggressive response scripts) which reflect past experiences and continue throughout development. As a person progresses into adulthood, these cognitive structures will influence his or her emotional and psychological state and affect their responses in a given social situation. This observation leads us to the necessity of placing ICT within the social domain and to question how it may be adapted to the treatment of impulsive aggression. We will present the theoretical premises of ICT as an intervention model and compare them with those of the SIP model of impulsive aggression. Thereafter, this will allow us to identify possible options of ways to adapt ICT to the treatment of impulsive aggression.

4.1 Theoretical aspects of the ICT model of intervention and SIP model of impulsive aggression

There exist several interventions that aim to reduce aggressive behavior, from early intervention in children [93, 94] to comprehensive programs for nonclinical adults [95, 96], to programs specific to individuals with psychopathology [97, 98]. Intervention programs are usually multimodal and are composed of an education component [93], and modules that target self-control [99], cognitive distortion modification [91], emotional regulation strategies [100], and the involvement of a person's environment [93]. For its part, with the aim of reducing behaviors that may be harmful to a person's health, ICT has taken place within the context of appetitive behaviors such as abusive relationships with food or eating [101], alcohol [102], drugs [103], and tobacco [104]. For some individuals, these behaviors have a significant reward value [105]. Although not specifically aimed at aggressive behavior, ICT targets behaviors that share a common basis with aggressive behavior. Indeed, appetitive behaviors [105] and aggressive impulsive behaviors [106] are characterized by a deficit of inhibitory control. It is therefore reasonable to believe that ICT can serve as a complementary module to interventions that are usually offered for the treatment of impulsive aggression.

ICT refers to a category of interventions in the form of cognitive training which uses computer-based tasks, such as the stop-signal task or the go/no-go task, which requires motor control functions to either restrain an action or cancel an ongoing action [107]. This training aims to increase inhibitory control skills that regulate appetitive behaviors. It is postulated that obesity and substance abuse are caused both by a hyper-valuation of an appetitive stimulus and hypo-function of inhibition mechanisms [108]. The procedure generally involves training a person to initiate an inhibition response to an external stimulus that visually represents the appetitive stimulus (i.e. unhealthy food or beer images; [109]). Meta-analysis has demonstrated a significant effect of ICT in the reduction of appetitive behaviors, as measured in a laboratory setting (ad-libitum; [105]). For some behaviors, it has been demonstrated to have generalized positive effects on the quality of a person's daily life (e.g., food intake; [110]). However, this has not been demonstrated for all behaviors (e.g., alcohol consumption; [107, 111]). This result supports the need to adapt ICT to the nature of certain impulsive behaviors. One of the mechanisms of action postulated to account for the effects of ICT is the creation of a bottom-up association between the appetitive stimulus and the inhibitory response that bypasses the need for a more general inhibitory control [101, 112].

Although inhibitory control is an important part of the intervention to reduce impulsive aggression behavior, several determinants are not accounted for within an ICT-based intervention model. At the level of situational determinants, the aggressive response may occur as a result of an external stimulus, such as a social provocation, but it may also occur as a result of an internal stimulus. Internal stimuli include the person's cognitions and emotions. Among cognitive determinants, for instance, when following an ambiguous social provocation, the interpretation that the other person has hostile intentions can lead to aggressive behavior [85]. Among emotional determinants, anger is well known as an internal state that can lead to reactive aggression [113]. However, it can be claimed that many other negative affective states, such as anxiety [114] or sadness [115], can also serve as an internal trigger for aggression. It has been observed that certain thoughts or strong emotions can affect the information processes of a person in a social situation [90]. The person's processing of information becomes incomplete or erroneous, and this increases the risk that the person will respond aggressively [116]. Moreover, negative feedback from the social environment in response to aggressive behavior can maintain those erroneous cognitions and intensify the negative affect of the aggressive person [13]. Interventions resulting from the SIP model are therefore intended to improve the accuracy and depth of a person's information processing ability. It also actively integrates the person's environment, which enriches positive social experiences that will ultimately change the way the person perceives the world and processes social information [117]. **Table 1** summarizes the main theoretical differences between the ICT and the SIP model of aggression.

4.2 Two-person neuropsychology

In terms of their theoretical premises, the ICT model and the SIP model may seem, at first glance, to be incompatible. However, we believe that it is possible to adapt ICT-based interventions to include the social domain. With this aim, we propose a novel approach to intervention for impulsive aggression, and consider a perspective based on two-person neuropsychology. Inspired by the two-person psychology approach, we will use the expression "two-person neuropsychology" in two ways. First, it refers to the idea that impulsive aggression occurs in the social domain and that neuropsychological interventions should aim to improve social information processes. The second meaning pertains to the transformation of cognitive structures within an individual with impulsive aggression, which we believe *requires* input from the other. According to SIP models of aggression, a distinction is made between two distinct components—"online situation-specific" and "offline person-specific" [117]. With "two-person neuropsychology," the first part would involve interventions that target the cognitive processes which take place in specific social situations, whereas the second part refers to interventions which target stable cognitive structures of the person.

4.3 Implementation intention strategy in support of ICT on cognitive processes

For individuals who are habitually aggressive, it has been shown that their social information cognitive processing is dysfunctional and influenced by erroneous cognitive structures [118]. In other words, the information being processed is

	ICT model	SIP model
Postulated causal mechanisms	Hyper-valuation of appetitive stimulus, stimulus reward and reward sensitivity Temporary lessening of inhibition function, which increases in response to an appetitive stimulus	Incomplete or erroneous social information processing Hostile cognitive structures that may interact with deficient executive functions (which include inhibition)
Triggers	External stimulus (i.e. smelling and/or viewing food or alcohol)	External (i.e., social provocation) and internal (i.e., negative affective state, such as anger) stimulus
Behavioral Maintenance Factors	Reward value of the appetitive stimulus	Negative social feedback
Postulated mechanisms of action	Top-down inhibitory control skill Automatic bottom-up association (stimulus-stop) Devaluation of stimulus, which follows the inhibition of stimulus	More accurate and in-depth social information processing Positive social feedback from appropriate social interactions

Table 1.
Comparison between the ICT and the SIP model of aggression.

largely based on pre-existing cognitive structures rather than on actual cues that are present in the social situation [13]. These structures lead to an automatic processing of the situation, which prevents the person from processing other relevant information which may be helpful in deciding the appropriate course of action in a given social situation [16]. Therefore, there is a link between a social situation and a cognitive process that appears conditioned by past experiences [119]. For example, a person who has been exposed to hostile situations in different social contexts during his or her development will be inclined to encode hostile information to the detriment of other non-hostile cues. Over time, this process becomes spontaneous and automatic [12]. For this reason, we believe that it is necessary to *disengage* the aggressive person from his erroneous cognitive processes, and help him or her to develop new associations between the same social situation and a new cognitive process. Given that ICT uses an external stimulus, and the automatic response which is targeted during training involves motor function, we recommended finding a comparable therapeutic strategy that would broaden ICT intervention targets. We feel that implementation intentions can serve this purpose. "Implementation intentions" is a self-regulation strategy that aims to help a person achieve their goal by implementing a series of behavioral steps. This includes (1) ensuring that behaviors are put in place in a specific situation, (2) these behaviors are designed to help the person achieve a desired goal which is planned in advance, and (3) the behaviors should take place automatically as soon as the situation is met [120–123]. This technique is based on an "if-then" contingency, where "if" represents the situation and "then" represents the response. The advantage of implementation intentions in relation to ICT is that the situation can be both external and internal, and the response can be modified and improved at any stage in the cognitive processing of social information. Also, this technique does not require lengthy training. For the most part, the focus is on verbalization and visualization of a plan. During these verbalization/visualization sessions, the person determines precisely all the elements of the situation which afford an opportunity to execute the plan. They also determine how they will act or respond cognitively in this particular situation. This strategy makes it possible to create new associations between a stimulus and a response, and in this respect, it appears compatible with one of the postulated mechanisms of action of ICT (e.g., creation of automatic bottom-up association). This association circumvents the necessity to make use of a general inhibitory control skill because the will of the person is delegated to the situation. Once established, such an association happens automatically (or quickly), efficiently, and without awareness. Also, because it is determined and planned in advance, the "if-then" plan represents an action restraint in which the decision to inhibit is made from the onset. As such, it is not an action cancelation, whereby the decision to inhibit occurs *after* implementation of the dominant response. This allows for cognitive processes to be similar to those running during a go/no-go task—the task that appears to be the most effective among ICT tasks [124].

4.4 Adaptation of ICT applied to impulsive aggression

Applied to impulsive aggression, the first step in implementing intentions would be to make an assessment of the person who is impulsively aggressive, and determine whether there are steps in the cognitive processing of social information which may be contributing to their aggressive behaviors. Subsequently, one can imagine that it is possible to plan if-then-type strategies for the step that is in question. Given that erroneous cognitive processing related to impulsive aggression mostly concerns the first steps in SIP [116, 117], the following discussion will be applied to the encoding, interpreting, and goal selecting processes.

Imagine the following social situation: you are at work and you receive a comment from one of your colleagues about your work. Based on an ICT model of intervention, this (or a similar situation) could make use of computer tasks during the training phase. At the level of the encoding step, the task could be similar to a dot-probe task [125], which is often used in research to measure attentional biases toward hostile cues in an aggressive person. The task is to present a pair of faces (both hostile and neutral) above and below a central point, which is followed by an arrow that points to the right or left in the upper or lower part of the screen. After viewing the presented cue, the person must indicate as quickly as possible in which direction the arrow was pointing. A hostile attentional bias is characterized by a shorter reaction time for arrows that appear where an angry face was presented, as compared to where a neutral face was presented. With the help of implementation intentions, a person might want to develop an if-then plan to encode more non-hostile cues into a situation where they receive feedback from a colleague. This plan would aim to create a new association between "a colleague made a comment about my work" and the attention directed toward non-hostile cues, such as "my colleague's facial expression." More specifically, during the training with the dot-probe task, the implementation intentions would aim at encoding non-hostile faces such as, "When the pair of faces appears on the screen, I will only pay attention to the neutral face." Such training could be generalized thereafter to real-life situations (e.g., "When my colleague makes a comment about my work, I will try to pay attention to his facial expression and see if he is *actually* criticizing me").

At the level of interpretation, the task could be an adaption of the "Hostile Expectancy Violation Paradigm" [126, 127], which involves a written scenario containing initial sentences that are used to establish a hostile versus non-hostile context, during which a character simultaneously commits an ambiguous behavior directed at the reader. These sentences are then followed with a third sentence that ends with a word informing the reader of the nature of the character's underlying intention for his or her behavior. The person would then be asked to guess the intention of the character before the presentation of the last word. Following a non-hostile context, a hostile interpretation of the character's ambiguous behavior would indicate a hostile attributional bias. With the help of implementation intentions, a person might want to develop a plan in order to interpret a colleague's comment about their work in a non-hostile manner. More specifically, during the training with the Hostile Expectancy Violation Paradigm, the implementation intentions would aim at interpreting non-hostile intention behind behaviors such as "When I read the intention sentence in which the last word reveals the intention of the character, I will think about a word that refers to a non-hostile intention". Again, such a training could be generalized thereafter to real-life situations (e.g., "When my colleague makes a comment about my work, I will try to think that my colleague did not make the comment with malicious intent").

Finally, in terms of goal selection and the emotions that accompany it, one can imagine that ideally, the plan is that the person does not act aggressively before the negative emotion has lessened. With the help of implementation intentions, a person might want to develop a plan to stop an impulsive behavior while experiencing a strong negative emotion. More specifically, during the training with the Hostile Expectancy Violation Paradigm (or other similar scenarios whereby a person could be asked to imagine his or her emotional response following a social provocation), the implementation intentions would aim to execute alternative behaviors to anger outbursts, such as "When I read the social provocation and I imagine that I feel anger toward the character, I will stop my reaction, breathe deeply and assess my level of anger. I will continue breathing or leave the place if my anger is still high." Again, such training could be generalized to real-life situations (e.g., "When my colleague makes a comment about my work, I will stop my reaction, breathe, assess my anger on a scale, and then wait until my anger has diminished before responding to my colleague").

4.5 Long-term interventions on hostile cognitive structures

We end this section with interventions that target the cognitive structures of aggressive individuals. We believe that only positive interactions with others or mid- to long-term psychotherapy can gradually change these relatively stable cognitive structures. In addition to cognitive therapy [128], several psychotherapy approaches have been proven effective in helping aggressive persons via the transformation of their mental structures. In order to prevent an impulsive behavioral response to an unconditioned experienced emotion, some interventions are designed to help individuals with mental elaboration (symbolization) of the emotional experience instead of acting out the emotion. The mental elaboration of the emotional experience makes the experience more tolerable and facilitates the development of more complex cognitive structures [129]. Other approaches aim to make individuals aware of their inner relational world, which influences their perceptions of people and the way they feel and relate to them [130]. When considering all the factors that are at play in an individual's mental life, we discover a multitude of social motivations that can contribute to acts of aggression, as well as psychological issues that may be associated with these behaviors [131]. A better self-awareness of these motivations and psychological issues could help aggressive persons transform their social cognitive structures. Finally, it is recommended that these interventions be accompanied by the development of positive relationships in real life. Marriage, family, or interpersonal therapies can support this goal, and new positive social interactions and relationships are expected to help change existing maladaptive hostile cognitive structures.

5. Conclusion

We have demonstrated the importance of social determinants in the development of hostile cognitive structures and the lack of inhibition in children. We have also demonstrated the cerebral connectivity underlying aggression in adults and its influence on the processing of social information. This has prompted us to want to adapt ICT and incorporate social cognition into its scope, which has thus far remained limited to the domain of motor control. We have proposed that implementation intentions strategy represents an intervention that is promising in achieving this goal. We believe that ICT adapted to the social field represents a promising therapeutic avenue to help people who suffer from impulsive aggression. However, this chapter is only a first step in this direction. We hope that this chapter can shed light on the issue of ICT in the treatment of impulsive aggression, and that it can stimulate both a theoretical debate and the realization of empirical study on the effectiveness of ICT in the treatment of impulsive aggression. On a daily basis, humans are in continual interaction with each other. There is little doubt that society would greatly benefit from interventions that are based on a better understanding of how internal knowledge structures serve as cognitive control mechanisms that perpetuate a cycle of impulsively aggressive behaviors.

Author details

J. Gagnon[1,2,3*], J.E. Quansah[1,2,3] and W.S. Kim[1,2,3]

1 Department of Psychology, University of Montréal, Canada

2 Centre for Interdisciplinary Research in Rehabilitation of Greater Montreal (CRIR), Montreal, Canada

3 Laboratoire d'Électrophysiologie en Neuroscience Sociale (LENS), Department of Psychology, University of Montreal, Canada

*Address all correspondence to: jean.gagnon@umontreal.ca

References

[1] Houston RJ et al. Neurobiological correlates and clinical implications of aggressive subtypes. Journal of Forensic Neuropsychology. 2003;**3**:67-87

[2] Parrott DJ, Zeichner A, Evces M. Effect of trait anger on cognitive processing of emotional stimuli. Journal of General Psychology. 2005;**132**(1):67-80

[3] Krug E et al. World Report on Violence and Health. Geneva: World Health Organization; 2002

[4] Stanford MS, Greve KW, Dickens TJ. Irritability and impulsiveness: Relationship to self-reported impulsive aggression. Personality and Individual Differences. 1995;**19**(5):757-760

[5] Gottlieb RM. Classical psychoanalysis. In: Textbook of Psychoanalysis. Washington, DC, USA: American Psychiatric Publishing; 2012. pp. 155-169

[6] Jacobs TJ. Countertransference past and present: A review of the concept. International Journal of Psychoanalysis. 1999;**80**:575-594

[7] Brown LJ. Transformational Processes. In: Legorreta G, editor. Clinical Psychoanalysis. New York, N.Y.: Routledge; 2019

[8] Criss MM et al. Family adversity, positive peer relationships, and children's externalizing behavior: A longitudinal perspective on risk and resilience. Child Development. 2002;**73**(4):1220-1237

[9] Barnow S, Freyberger H-J. The family environment in early life and aggressive behavior in adolescents and young adults. In: Mattson MP, editor. Neurobiology of Aggression: Understanding and Preventing Violence. Totowa, NJ: Humana Press; 2003. pp. 213-229

[10] Malinosky-Rummell R, Hansen DJ. Long-term consequences of childhood physical abuse. Psychological Bulletin. 1993;**114**(1):68-79

[11] Crick NR, Dodge KA. A review and reformulation of social information-processing mechanisms in children's social adjustment. Psychological Bulletin. 1994;**115**(1):74-101

[12] Huesmann LR. An information processing model for the development of aggression. Aggressive Behavior. 1988;**14**(1):13-24

[13] Anderson CA, Bushman BJ. Human aggression. Annual Review of Psychology. 2002;**53**(1):27-51

[14] Dodge KA. Translational science in action: Hostile attributional style and the development of aggressive behavior problems. Development and Psychopathology. 2006;**18**(3):791-814

[15] Higgins ET. Personality, social psychology, and person-situation relations: Standards and knowledge activation as a common language. In: Handbook of Personality: Theory and Research. New York, NY, USA: The Guilford Press; 1990. pp. 301-338

[16] Todorov A, Bargh JA. Automatic sources of aggression. Aggression and Violent Behavior. 2002;**7**(1):53-68

[17] Higgins ET. Knowledge activation: Accessibility, applicability, and salience. In: Social Psychology: Handbook of Basic Principles. New York, NY, USA: The Guilford Press; 1996. pp. 133-168

[18] Nasby W, Hayden B, DePaulo BM. Attributional bias among aggressive boys to interpret unambiguous

social stimuli as displays of hostility. Journal of Abnormal Psychology. 1980;**89**(3):459-468

[19] Dodge KA, Coie JD. Social-information-processing factors in reactive and proactive aggression in children's peer groups. Journal of Personality and Social Psychology. 1987;**53**(6):1146-1158

[20] Bushman BJ. Violent media and hostile appraisals: A meta-analytic review. Aggressive Behavior. 2016;**42**(6):605-613

[21] Anderson CA et al. The influence of media violence on youth. Psychological Science in the Public Interest. 2003;**4**(3):81-110

[22] Berkowitz L. Aggression: Its Causes, Consequences, and Control. New York, NY, England: Mcgraw-Hill Book Company; 1993. 485p

[23] Fiske ST, Taylor SE. Social Cognition. 2nd ed. New York, NY, England: Mcgraw-Hill Book Company; 1991. 717p

[24] Bushman BJ, Huesmann LR. Short-term and long-term effects of violent media on aggression in children and adults. Archives of Pediatrics and Adolescent Medicine. 2006;**160**(4):348-352

[25] Burks VS et al. Internal representational models of peers: Implications for the development of problematic behavior. Developmental Psychology. 1999;**35**(3):802-810

[26] Huesmann LR, Guerra NG. Children's normative beliefs about aggression and aggressive behavior. Journal of Personality and Social Psychology. 1997;**72**(2):408-419

[27] Guerra NG, Huesmann LR, Hanish L. The role of normative beliefs in children's social behavior. In: Social Development. Thousand Oaks, CA, USA: Sage Publications, Inc; 1995. pp. 140-158

[28] Asarnow JR, Callan JW. Boys with peer adjustment problems: Social cognitive processes. Journal of Consulting and Clinical Psychology. 1985;**53**(1):80-87

[29] Crick NR, Ladd GW. Children's perceptions of the outcomes of social strategies: Do the ends justify being mean? Developmental Psychology. 1990;**26**(4):612-620

[30] Dodge KA et al. Social competence in children. Monographs of the Society for Research in Child Development. 1986;**51**(2):1-85

[31] Perry DG, Perry LC, Rasmussen P. Cognitive social learning mediators of aggression. Child Development. 1986;**57**(3):700-711

[32] Quiggle NL et al. Social information processing in aggressive and depressed children. Child Development. 1992;**63**(6):1305-1320

[33] Crick N, Dodge K. Children's perceptions of peer entry and conflict situations: Social strategies, goals, and outcome expectations. In: Social Competence in Developmental Perspective. New York, NY, USA: Kluwer Academic/Plenum Publishers; 1989. pp. 396-399

[34] Musher-Eizenman DR et al. Social-cognitive mediators of the relation of environmental and emotion regulation factors to Children's aggression. Aggressive Behavior. 2004;**30**(5):389-408

[35] Miller-Johnson S et al. Peer rejection and aggression and early starter models of conduct disorder. Journal of Abnormal Child Psychology. 2002;**30**(3):217-230

[36] Baddeley A. Working Memory. New York, NY, USA: Clarendon Press/ Oxford University Press; 1986. 289p

[37] Séguin JR, Zelazo PD. Executive function in early physical aggression. In: Developmental Origins of Aggression. New York, NY, USA: The Guilford Press; 2005. pp. 307-329

[38] Anderson CA, Bushman BJ. Media violence and the general aggression model. Journal of Social Issues. 2018;**74**(2):386-413

[39] Bartholow BD. The aggressive brain: Insights from neuroscience. Current Opinion in Psychology. 2018;**19**:60-64

[40] Hoaken PN, Shaughnessy VK, Pihl R. Executive cognitive functioning and aggression: Is it an issue of impulsivity? Aggressive Behavior: Official Journal of the International Society for Research on Aggression. 2003;**29**(1):15-30

[41] Curtin JJ, Fairchild BA. Alcohol and cognitive control: Implications for regulation of behavior during response conflict. Journal of Abnormal Psychology. 2003;**112**(3):424

[42] Giancola PR, Zeichner A. Neuropsychological performance on tests of frontal-lobe functioning and aggressive behavior in men. Journal of Abnormal Psychology. 1994;**103**(4):832

[43] Tonnaer F, Cima M, Arntz A. Executive (dys) functioning and impulsivity as possible vulnerability factors for aggression in forensic patients. The Journal of Nervous and Mental Disease. 2016;**204**(4):280-286

[44] Cima M, Raine A. Distinct characteristics of psychopathy relate to different subtypes of aggression. Personality and Individual Differences. 2009;**47**(8):835-840

[45] Miyake A et al. The unity and diversity of executive functions and their contributions to complex "frontal lobe" tasks: A latent variable analysis. Cognitive Psychology. 2000;**41**(1):49-100

[46] De Bellis MD. Developmental traumatology: The psychobiological development of maltreated children and its implications for research, treatment, and policy. Development and Psychopathology. 2001;**13**(3):539-564

[47] De Bellis MD. The psychobiology of neglect. Child Maltreatment. 2005;**10**(2):150-172

[48] Hart H, Rubia K. Neuroimaging of child abuse: A critical review. Frontiers in Human Neuroscience. 2012;**6**:52

[49] Hughes C, Graham A. Executive function in childhood: Development and disorder. In: Oates J, Grayson A, editors. Cognitive and Language Development in Children. Oxford: Blackwell Publishing Ltd; 2004. pp. 205-230

[50] McCrory E, De Brito SA, Viding E. The impact of childhood maltreatment: A review of neurobiological and genetic factors. Frontiers in Psychiatry. 2011;**2**:48

[51] Teicher MH, Anderson CM, Polcari A. Childhood maltreatment is associated with reduced volume in the hippocampal subfields CA3, dentate gyrus, and subiculum. Proceedings of the National Academy of Sciences of the United States of America. 2012;**109**(9):E563-E572

[52] Johnson MH. Interactive specialization: A domain-general framework for human functional brain development? Developmental Cognitive Neuroscience. 2011;**1**(1):7-21

[53] Teicher MH et al. The neurobiological consequences of early stress and childhood maltreatment.

Neuroscience and Biobehavioral Reviews. 2003;**27**(1-2):33-44

[54] Goldweber A et al. Examining factors associated with (in)stability in social information processing among urban school children: A latent transition analytic approach. Journal of Clinical Child and Adolescent Psychology. 2011;**40**(5):715-729

[55] van Nieuwenhuijzen M et al. Impulse control and aggressive response generation as predictors of aggressive behaviour in children with mild intellectual disabilities and borderline intelligence. Journal of Intellectual Disability Research. 2009;**53**(3):233-242

[56] van Nieuwenhuijzen M, Vriens A. (social) Cognitive skills and social information processing in children with mild to borderline intellectual disabilities. Research in Developmental Disabilities. 2012;**33**(2):426-434

[57] Van Nieuwenhuijzen M et al. Executive functions and social information processing in adolescents with severe behavior problems. Child Neuropsychology. 2017;**23**(2):228-241

[58] Ellis ML, Weiss B, Lochman JE. Executive functions in children: Associations with aggressive behavior and appraisal processing. Journal of Abnormal Child Psychology. 2009;**37**(7):945-956

[59] Frankenhuis WE, de Weerth C. Does early-life exposure to stress shape or impair cognition? Current Directions in Psychological Science. 2013;**22**(5):407-412

[60] Mittal C et al. Cognitive adaptations to stressful environments: When childhood adversity enhances adult executive function. Journal of Personality and Social Psychology. 2015;**109**(4):604-621

[61] Brezina T, Tekin E, Topalli V. "Might not be a tomorrow": A multimethods approach to anticipated early death and youth crime. Criminology. 2009;**47**(4):1091-1129

[62] Fawcett TW, McNamara JM, Houston AI. When is it adaptive to be patient? A general framework for evaluating delayed rewards. Behavioural Processes. 2012;**89**(2):128-136

[63] Daly M, Wilson M. Carpe diem: Adaptation and devaluing the future. The Quarterly Review of Biology. 2005;**80**(1):55-60

[64] DeWall CN et al. Violence restrained: Effects of self-regulation and its depletion on aggression. Journal of Experimental Social Psychology. 2007;**43**(1):62-76

[65] Nelson RJ, Trainor BC. Neural mechanisms of aggression. Nature Reviews Neuroscience. 2007;**8**(7):536

[66] Damasio H et al. The return of Phineas gage: Clues about the brain from the skull of a famous patient. Science. 1994;**264**(5162):1102-1105

[67] van Honk J et al. Socially explosive minds: The triple imbalance hypothesis of reactive aggression. Journal of Personality. 2010;**78**(1):67-94

[68] Coccaro EF et al. Corticolimbic function in impulsive aggressive behavior. Biological Psychiatry. 2011;**69**(12):1153-1159

[69] Lane SD, Kjome KL, Moeller FG. Neuropsychiatry of aggression. Neurologic Clinics. 2011;**29**(1):49

[70] Meijers J et al. Prison brain? Executive dysfunction in prisoners. Frontiers in psychology. 2015;**6**:43

[71] Fanning JR et al. Neural correlates of aggressive behavior in real time: A

review of fMRI studies of laboratory reactive aggression. Current Behavioral Neuroscience Reports. 2017;**4**(2):138-150

[72] Lieberman MD, Eisenberger NI. Pains and pleasures of social life. Science. 2009;**323**(5916):890-891

[73] Chester DS et al. Monoamine oxidase A (MAOA) genotype predicts greater aggression through impulsive reactivity to negative affect. Behavioural Brain Research. 2015;**283**:97-101

[74] Coccaro EF et al. Amygdala and orbitofrontal reactivity to social threat in individuals with impulsive aggression. Biological psychiatry. 2007;**62**(2):168-178

[75] Fettich KC et al. Emotion regulation deficits in intermittent explosive disorder. Aggressive Behavior. 2015;**41**(1):25-33

[76] Puhalla AA et al. Negative urgency and reward/punishment sensitivity in intermittent explosive disorder. Journal of Affective Disorders. 2016;**201**:8-14

[77] Nomura M et al. Functional association of the amygdala and ventral prefrontal cortex during cognitive evaluation of facial expressions primed by masked angry faces: An event-related fMRI study. NeuroImage. 2004;**21**(1):352-363

[78] Chester DS, et al. Neural correlates of intertemporal choice in aggressive behavior. Aggressive behavior. 2019

[79] Leary MR, Twenge JM, Quinlivan E. Interpersonal rejection as a determinant of anger and aggression. Personality and Social Psychology Review. 2006;**10**(2):111-132

[80] General, US Surgeon. Youth Violence: A Report of the Surgeon General. Washington, DC: US Department of Health and Human Services, Office of the Secretary, Office of Public Health and Science, Office of the Surgeon General; 2001

[81] Baumeister RF, Twenge JM, Nuss CK. Effects of social exclusion on cognitive processes: Anticipated aloneness reduces intelligent thought. Journal of Personality and Social Psychology. 2002;**83**(4):817

[82] Achterberg M et al. Control your anger! The neural basis of aggression regulation in response to negative social feedback. Social Cognitive and Affective Neuroscience. 2016;**11**(5):712-720

[83] Camodeca M, Goossens FA. Aggression, social cognitions, anger and sadness in bullies and victims. Journal of Child Psychology and Psychiatry. 2005;**46**(2):186-197

[84] Dodge KA, Coie JD, Lynam D. Aggression and antisocial behavior in youth. In: Handbook of Child Psychology. Vol. 3. 2007

[85] De Castro BO et al. Hostile attribution of intent and aggressive behavior: A meta-analysis. Child Development. 2002;**73**(3):916-934

[86] Lansford JE et al. Developmental trajectories of externalizing and internalizing behaviors: Factors underlying resilience in physically abused children. Development and Psychopathology. 2006;**18**(1):35-55

[87] Dodge KA, Pettit GS. A biopsychosocial model of the development of chronic conduct problems in adolescence. Developmental Psychology. 2003;**39**(2):349

[88] Guerra NG, Rowell Huesmann L, Spindler A. Community violence exposure, social cognition, and aggression among urban elementary school children. Child Development. 2003;**74**(5):1561-1576

[89] Repple J et al. From provocation to aggression: The neural network. BMC Neuroscience. 2017;**18**(1):73

[90] Lemerise E, Arsenio W. An integrated model of emotion processes and cognition in social information processing. Child Development. 2000;**71**:107-118

[91] Hudley C, Graham S. An attributional intervention to reduce peer-directed aggression among African-American boys. Child Development. 1993;**64**(1):124-138

[92] Huesmann LR, Eron LD. Cognitive processes and the persistence of aggressive behavior. Aggressive Behavior. 1984;**10**(3):243-251

[93] Barkley RA et al. Multi-method psycho-educational intervention for preschool children with disruptive behavior: Preliminary results at post-treatment. Journal of Child Psychology and Psychiatry, and Allied Disciplines. 2000;**41**(3):319-332

[94] Groark CJ et al. Improvements in early care in Russian orphanages and their relationship to observed behaviors. Infant Mental Health Journal. 2005;**26**(2):96-109

[95] Guerra NG, Slaby RG. Evaluative factors in social-problem solving by aggressive boys. Journal of Abnormal Child Psychology. 1989;**17**:277-289

[96] Siddle R, Jones F, Awenat F. Group cognitive behaviour therapy for anger: A pilot study. Behavioural and Cognitive Psychotherapy. 2003;**31**(1):69-83

[97] Ahmed A et al. Cognitive training for impulsive aggression in schizophrenia. Schizophrenia Bulletin. 2019;**45**:S271-S272

[98] Lindenmayer JP et al. Cognitive training for social cognition in impulsive aggression in schizophrenia. Schizophrenia Bulletin. 2019;**45**:S217-S218

[99] Gallo IS et al. Downregulation of anger by mental contrasting with implementation intentions (MCII). Frontiers in Psychology. 2018;**9**:1838

[100] Franco C et al. Effect of a mindfulness training program on the impulsivity and aggression levels of adolescents with behavioral problems in the classroom. Frontiers in Psychology. 2016;**7**:1385

[101] Oomen D et al. Beating uncontrolled eating: Training inhibitory control to reduce food intake and food cue sensitivity. Appetite. 2018;**131**:73-83

[102] Di Lemma LCG, Field M. Cue avoidance training and inhibitory control training for the reduction of alcohol consumption: A comparison of effectiveness and investigation of their mechanisms of action. Psychopharmacology. 2017;**234**(16):2489-2498

[103] Alcorn JL et al. A pilot investigation of acute inhibitory control training in cocaine users. Drug and Alcohol Dependence. 2017;**174**:145-149

[104] Adams S et al. Resisting the urge to smoke: Inhibitory control training in cigarette smokers. Royal Society Open Science. 2017;**4**(8):170045

[105] Jones A et al. Inhibitory control training for appetitive behaviour change: A meta-analytic investigation of mechanisms of action and moderators of effectiveness. Appetite. 2016;**97**:16-28

[106] Kraemer UM et al. The role of executive functions in the control of aggressive behavior. Frontiers in Psychology. 2011;**2**:152

[107] Jones A et al. A randomized controlled trial of inhibitory control training for the reduction of alcohol

consumption in problem drinkers. Journal of Consulting and Clinical Psychology. 2018;**86**(12):991-1004

[108] Volkow ND et al. Overlapping neuronal circuits in addiction and obesity: Evidence of systems pathology. Philosophical Transactions of the Royal Society, B: Biological Sciences. 2008;**363**(1507):3191-3200

[109] Jones A, Field M. The effects of Cue-specific inhibition training on alcohol consumption in heavy social drinkers. Experimental and Clinical Psychopharmacology. 2013;**21**(1):8-16

[110] Forman EM et al. Mindful decision making and inhibitory control training as complementary means to decrease snack consumption. Appetite. 2016;**103**:176-183

[111] Allom V, Mullan B. Two inhibitory control training interventions designed to improve eating behaviour and determine mechanisms of change. Appetite. 2015;**89**:282-290

[112] Veling H et al. What is trained during food go/no-go training? A review focusing on mechanisms and research agenda. Current Addiction Reports. 2017;**4**(1):35-41

[113] Wilkowski BM, Robinson MD. The anatomy of anger: An integrative cognitive model of trait anger and reactive aggression. Journal of Personality. 2010;**78**(1):9-38

[114] Hawkins KA, Cougle JR. Anger problems across the anxiety disorders: Findings from a population-based study. Depression and Anxiety. 2011;**28**(2):145-152

[115] Smith HL et al. Hostile interpretation bias in depression. Journal of Affective Disorders. 2016;**203**:9-13

[116] Crick NR, Dodge KA. A review and reformulation of social-information processing mechanisms in children's development. Psychological Bulletin. 1994;**115**:74-101

[117] de Castro BO, van Dijk A. It is gonna end up with a fight anyway. In: Lochman JE, Matthys W, editors. The Wiley Handbook of Disruptive and Impulsive-Control Disorders. Hoboken, N.J: John Wiley and sons Ltd; 2018

[118] Calvete E, Orue I. Social information processing as a mediator between cognitive schemas and aggressive behavior in adolescents. Journal of Abnormal Child Psychology. 2012;**40**(1):105-117

[119] Lochman JE, Dodge KA. Distorted perceptions in dyadic interactions of aggressive and nonaggressive boys: Effects of prior expectations, context, and boys' age. Development and Psychopathology. 1998;**10**(3):495-512

[120] Gollwitzer PM, Sheeran P. Implementation intentions and goal achievement: A meta-analysis of effects and processes. Advances in experimental social psychology. 2006;**38**(6):69-119

[121] Gollwitzer PM. Weakness of the will: Is a quick fix possible? Motivation and Emotion. 2014;**38**:305-322

[122] Gollwitzer PM. Implementation intentions: Strong effects of simple plans. American Psychologist. 1999;**54**(7):493-503

[123] Sheeran P, Webb TL, Gollwitzer PM. The interplay between goal intentions and implementation intentions. Personality and Social Psychology Bulletin. 2005;**31**(1):87-98

[124] Allom V, Mullan B, Hagger M. Does inhibitory control training improve health behaviour? A meta-analysis. Health Psychology Review. 2016;**10**(2):168-186

[125] MacLeod C et al. Selective attention and emotional vulnerability: Assessing the causal basis of their assocation through the experimental manipulation of attentional Bais. Journal of Abnormal Psychology. 2002;**111**(1):107-123

[126] Gagnon J et al. Neural mechanisms underlying attribution of hostile intention in nonaggressive individuals: An ERP study. International Journal of Psychophysiology. 2016;**110**:153-162

[127] Gagnon J et al. An ERP study on hostile attribution bias in aggressive and nonaggressive individuals. Aggressive Behavior. 2017;**43**:217-229

[128] Beck AT et al. Cognitive Therapy of Personality Disorders. 2nd ed. New York: The Guilford Press; 2004

[129] Bateman A et al. A randomised controlled trial of mentalization-based treatment versus structured clinical management for patients with comorbid borderline personality disorder and antisocial personality disorder. BMC Psychiatry. 2016;**16**:304

[130] Kernberg OF. An overview of the treatment of sever-narcissist pathology. International Journal of Psychoanalysis. 2014;**95**(5):865-888

[131] Yakeley J, Meloy JR. Understanding violence: Does psychoanalytic thinking matter? Aggression and Violent Behavior. 2012;**17**(3):229-239